The
SLOW
DOWN
DIET

"Rushed, mindless eating creates weight-loss resistance. *The Slow Down Diet* provides an easy-to-apply, work-anywhere, 8-week plan that helps you relax, reduce stress, and savor every mouthful while burning fat and optimizing health."

J. J. VIRGIN, NUTRITIONIST AND AUTHOR
OF THE BESTSELLING *JJ VIRGIN'S SUGAR IMPACT DIET*

"I love Marc David's *The Slow Down Diet*—it is joyfully entertaining, educational, and provides clear, practical steps to not only help people with their weight loss goals but also with their quest to be healthier and happier."

MICHAEL T. MURRAY, ND, COAUTHOR OF
THE ENCYCLOPEDIA OF NATURAL MEDICINE

"Marc David is a master of transformation. He helps us see the underlying reasons *why* we eat the way we do and lovingly helps us move through the behaviors that don't serve us. In a world of fad diets and insane trends, Marc's teachings are timeless, relevant, and effective. Slow down and enjoy a book that'll change your life."

PEDRAM SHOJAI, OMD,
FILMMAKER AND FOUNDER OF WELL.ORG

"Finally, a diet book that works! *The Slow Down Diet* by Marc David is a classic. It is a book that will take you from where you are to where you want to be. A must read for anyone looking to achieve a higher health potential."

DR. FABRIZIO MANCINI, AUTHOR OF *THE POWER OF SELF-HEALING* AND MEDIA HEALTHY LIVING EXPERT

"*The Slow Down Diet* is a metabolic masterpiece integrating body, mind, and spiritual wisdom like only Marc David can do! An inspiring read for all those interested in nourishing a healthy, loving, and peaceful relationship with food."

KATHIE MADONNA SWIFT, M.S., RDN, LDN, FAND, AND COAUTHOR OF *THE SWIFT DIET: 4 WEEKS TO MEND THE BELLY, LOSE THE WEIGHT, AND GET RID OF THE BLOAT*

10TH ANNIVERSARY EDITION

The
SLOW
DOWN
DIET

Eating for Pleasure, Energy, and Weight Loss

MARC DAVID

Healing Arts Press
Rochester, Vermont • Toronto, Canada

Healing Arts Press
One Park Street
Rochester, Vermont 05767
www.InnerTraditions.com

Healing Arts Press is a division of Inner Traditions International

Note to the reader: This book is intended as an informational guide. The remedies, approaches, and techniques described herein are meant to supplement, and not to be a substitute for, professional medical care or treatment. They should not be used to treat a serious ailment without prior consultation with a qualified health care professional.

The Library of Congress has cataloged the earlier edition as follows:
David, Marc.
  The slow down diet : eating for pleasure, energy, and weight loss / Marc David.
    p. cm.
  Includes bibliographical references.
  ISBN 1-59477-060-3
  1. Nutrition. 2. Food habits. 3. Relaxation. I. Title.
  RA784.D375 2005
  613.2—dc22

                                                            2005000206

New edition ISBN 978-1-62055-508-8 (pbk) — ISBN 978-1-62055-509-5 (e-book)

Printed and bound in the United States by Versa Press, Inc.

10 9 8 7 6

Text design and layout by Rachel Goldenberg
This book was typeset in Garamond Premier Pro with Helvetica Neue and Agenda used as display typefaces

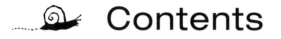 # Contents

Acknowledgments

A book is a very personal creation, yet anyone who has contributed to me or touched my life will somehow find their afterglow in these pages.

First and foremost, a special heartfelt and eternal thank you to my parents who've long since passed on, Sidney and Rachel. As the years move by, I'm astounded at how lucky and blessed I am to have had such loving and committed parents. Words are inadequate to say how much I've received from you. I hope my work continues to honor you both.

Next, my deepest respect and honor to all my ancestors and relations who've passed on, especially my grandparents—Charles and Molly Cohen and Jack and Esther Weinstein, Uncle Sid, Uncle Jerry, Uncle Eddy, and Aunt Sandy. Your love is forever imprinted in my psyche.

The late Douglas Brady was my best friend and soul brother. Thank you for all the ways you loved and supported me. I miss you dearly.

My family has been the most amazing springboard. My deepest love and appreciation goes out to my uncle Ronald Cohen, my aunt Ceil Sherry, Uncle David, and Aunt Bunny. My cousin, David Cohen, has deeply and abundantly fulfilled the role of the brother I never had, while Rusty Cohen has magically shown up as the special cousin I always wanted.

Much love to my family tribe who have been faithful and ever present: the Goldstones—Rhonda, Tony, Jonathan, and Andrew, we've had so many wonderful times together. Brad Cohen always inspires me simply by being Brad, generous and loving. Jeffrey Cohen always keeps me smiling and plotting my next move. Rick Cohen is my favorite alpha male and awes me with his huge heart. More Cohens to appreciate: Mitchell, Jason, Jodi, Brendan, Courtney, Matthew, and Ben.

I am blessed with some amazing friends in my life. Mark Hyman— thanks for being such a dear friend, powerful ally, soul brother, and intellectual co-conspirator. Gudni Gunnarsson has been a loving brother, mentor, and guide and always helps me return to my truest self. Pier Paolo de Angelis has been a special friend who helps me celebrate life to the fullest while remembering the deeper truths of who we are and why we're all here on Planet Earth. Jordan Blank has been my oldest friend and has been such a huge support and inspiration in so many ways. Thank you for being there.

More appreciation to those who've been so faithful and meaningful on my life's journey: Tom and Kathy Jackman, Dharani Burnham, Mark Kelso and Arti Ross-Kelso, Alexander Souri, John Dekadt, Michael Johnson, and Joan Berry. Toinette Lippe, my editor for my first book, Nourishing Wisdom, has always been such a big support and special angel.

A special thank you goes out to our amazing tribe of students, graduates, participants, fans, and staff of the Institute for the Psychology of Eating. When I founded the Institute I had no idea how it would grow and catch fire so swiftly. I'm honored to be part of this great mission together where we are forever changing the way the world understands food, body, and health.

My deep gratitude goes out to the staff, guests, and extended families of the Kripalu Center for Yoga and Health and Canyon Ranch in the Berkshires—two wonderfully bright lights in the world of healing and transformation that I've had the honor to be part of. Sonoma State University where I did my graduate work was a special place to educate both mind and soul.

There have been some very special luminaries in my life who have deeply influenced my work, my thinking, and my destiny. I owe so much to the late James Hillman—a man far ahead of his time in wisdom and insight. Thank you for awakening my mind. The late Gordon Tappan, my beloved professor and mentor, helped light a spark inside me. Ken Wilber has powerfully influenced my worldview and his brilliance informs my work. More important influencers in my life who live inside me include Robert Greenway, Rudolf Steiner, Martin Luther King, Robert Bly, Lao Tzu, Oscar Wilde, Jeff Bland, Carl Jung, Amrit Desai, Osho, Gerhart Schmidt, and Nikola Tesla.

For me, place has often been as special and necessary as people. Thank you to the Green River, Monument Mountain, Kennedy Park, Maui, Big Beach, Little Beach, Baldwin Beach, La Perouse, the Big Island, the Gunks, Hawk Meadow, Boulder, Buena Vista, Buckingham Park, Venice, Jacob's Pillow (for providing amazing dance), and of course, the place where all sentient life seems to be able to trace its roots—Brooklyn.

Nature is always my refuge. It never lies. Thanks especially to the dolphin and whale tribe who have magically allowed me in.

I'm so grateful to all the wonderful staff at Inner Traditions/Healing Arts Press, including Jon Graham, Susan Davidson, and Jeanie Levitan. Thanks for doing such great work in the world. I'm fortunate to have such a caring and amazing publishing house. Thanks as well to Ehud Sperling for creating such a wonderful company.

Emily Rosen, my brilliant and beautiful partner in life and in love, has been my muse and inspiration. She's the angel that stepped into my heart when I needed her most. I feel like the luckiest man in the world. Thanks for seeing me, for so many special times together, and for all the magic we share. Words could never express my deep love for you, and my appreciation for how you've forever transformed my world. And thank you for being an unstoppable force as the Director of the Institute for the Psychology of Eating, making it a shining light for so many people around the globe. Your efforts and smarts as a businesswoman and mission driven teacher, coach, and mentor are a wonder to witness and behold. I love you.

Lastly, my thanks to the Creator of All for a beautiful and crazy life and for sending down Skye, my special son, fellow rock collector, sports fanatic, and my favorite guy forever.

MARC DAVID
BOULDER, COLORADO
2015

Preface to the Tenth Anniversary Edition

Dear Reader,

I'm so honored to be celebrating and updating *The Slow Down Diet* for its tenth anniversary edition. These days most books never make it past a year on the shelves. I've made the commitment to write books on nutrition, eating psychology, and personal transformation that are timeless and truly meaningful. When it comes to these topics, I find that people are pretty hungry for both information *and* wisdom that makes a real difference.

The Slow Down Diet has been a life-changing book for so many people. I'm humbled by the extensive praise it's received and I'm thankful that it has found its way to so many of the people who need it most. I believe that if a book truly has value, then it grows wings of its own and is moved by an unseen power. *The Slow Down Diet* has certainly found a magic way to fly . . .

If you look around you, I think you'll notice that we live in a time of tremendous confusion around what to eat and what not to eat. The field of nutrition is filled with conflicting advice. At the same time there's an equal amount of pain and suffering when it comes to our relationship with food and body. Obesity is on the rise, along with increasing concerns around body image, overeating, binge eating, emotional eating, endless dieting, weight hate, and unwanted food habits.

Such food concerns rob of us of our personal power and stop of us from fulfilling our greatest potential. The problem is, so many of our dietary strategies are focused on pushing, forcing, over-exercising, under-eating, and hating the body into submission. After all, if we can speak enough negativity to ourselves about our own body and diet, then surely this will motivate us. The problem is though, it's impossible to go down a road of self-attack and self-hate and end up at a place of self-love. The journey informs the destination.

The Slow Down Diet offers an alternative way through. It's a book that's here to bring out the best of who we are as eaters. It's written to address head-on the challenges we face as human beings in navigating the uncertain terrain of nourishing the body. It's a book about food and body that's positive, uplifting, and heartfelt—while being fanatically results-oriented and firmly grounded in mind-body science.

I've been on a life-long mission to advance the fields of eating psychology and nutrition. For many years I worked in the supplement industry in product development and formulation, consulting with some of the biggest food, vitamin, drug, and media companies you've heard of. I've logged thousands of client hours over my thirty years in clinical practice, taught every kind of audience you can imagine, and used my own body as a laboratory. In short—I've covered as much turf as I could in the nutrition and health arena. I wrote my first book, *Nourishing Wisdom,* in 1990. That book has stayed in print for about twenty-five years and is considered a classic and groundbreaking work. I'm happy to say that *The Slow Down Diet* continues in that tradition.

Back in 2005 I had a traveling and teaching schedule that was way too busy. I was a single dad and wanted to stay put in one place and raise my son. I was also hearing an undeniable voice in my head telling me to start a teaching organization and get my work out there in a bigger way. Have you ever had that happen to you—the improbable or even otherworldly voice-in-the-head-thing telling you to do something that you know you have to do, but you know it won't be so easy? I resisted as best I could, but the voice in my head won out.

So I started the Institute for the Psychology of Eating, and it's grown to be an educational organization that's far surpassed what I thought possible. The Institute has a worldwide reach and features truly innovative and groundbreaking trainings for both professionals and the public that combine the psychology of eating with the science of nutrition. We literally have millions of followers, fans, and tribe members who all have a shared mission—to forever change the way the world understands food, body and health.

Much of the wisdom and the results-producing strategies that you'll find in this book are based upon the unique body of knowledge we teach at the Institute for the Psychology of Eating. I have the great privilege to train students to work with the most common and compelling eating challenges of our times—weight, body image, overeating, binge eating, emotional eating, endless dieting, and nutrition-related health challenges that have an emotional component such as digestion, fatigue, mood, immunity, and others.

And that's the essence of this book you're reading—an alternative approach to healing our relationship with food, body, planet, and soul.

I think what truly qualifies me to do this work is that I care in a deep way. I feel moved. For me, this work is a calling. The fields of eating psychology and nutrition have given so much to me personally and professionally that I want to give back as best I can. I want to live a life where I wake up feeling good in the morning because I do good work in the world that makes a real difference. I'm happy to say, mission accomplished.

I love seeing the magic that happens when someone's health and energy returns because they found the right nutritional or emotional course corrections. I love when people see their symptoms or ailments finally resolve themselves, when their eating challenges relax in a big way, and when people become vibrant and inspired enough that their well-nourished bodies now becomes vehicles to live a life that's meaningful.

The Slow Down Diet is my way of sharing with you some of the greatest lessons, tricks, and shortcuts I've learned in eating psychology and nutrition. It will likely go against much of what you've learned previously about eating healthy and losing weight. It will challenge some of the most cherished advice the experts have offered. It won't disfavor you with yet another dietary prescription that dictates precisely what to eat, when to eat it, and how much. Nor will it seduce you with a system that's difficult to follow and destined to fall by the wayside. Rather, this book will show you how to optimize metabolism no matter what you choose to eat.

And it will teach you how to access the wisdom of the greatest dietary authority on planet Earth: the nutritionist within you.

It's time to find real and lasting relief from our eating challenges, and to finally discover a relationship with food and body that's truly nourishing and empowering. If you've been trying to lighten your load by following all the latest diets but without any lasting success, this book will show you why and what to do about it. If you feel frustrated and confused by the news of all the conflicting nutrition systems that bombard the airwaves, these pages will provide the insights and relief you've been hoping for and that you well deserve. Ultimately, *The Slow Down Diet* will help bring the gifts of the soul into your dietary world and in doing so will awaken an inner fire that's the true source of our power.

Enjoy. A new metabolic you is about to be born . . .

Introduction

In Polynesian folklore, Maui is a demigod without equal; the beautiful Hawaiian island is named in his honor. A clever trickster with superhuman strength, Maui's most extraordinary and memorable exploit was his capture of the sun.

Soon after Maui raised up the sky to allow humans to walk upright and to clear the way for Sun to rise to an elevated position from the lower world, trouble began. Sun selfishly proceeded to race through the sky rather than arc across the heavens at a leisurely pace. This gave the people little time to fish, grow food, or dry their tapa cloth. They grew sick and unhappy.

With sage advice from his grandmother, Maui devised a plan to aid the suffering people. For many days he hid at the eastern end of the tallest volcano, Haleakala, and calculated Sun's daily path. He returned home to make sixteen strong ropes from his sister's hair as he prepared to use his legendary strength to lasso Sun.

The next morning, as Sun rose over Haleakala and began its self-indulgent flight across the sky, Maui grabbed the first ray to appear and tied it to a strong wiliwili tree. He soon had all sixteen rays secured.

Immobilized, Sun was at Maui's mercy and wisely agreed to a bargain. In exchange for his life, Sun promised to move slowly and thoughtfully across the sky, thus allowing the people the conditions for

1

nourishment and prosperity. They were so happy and Sun so honored that to this day Sun has kept his word.

It's no accident that the sun has become a symbol of metabolism. It is the ultimate source of energy on planet Earth. We acknowledge it by referring to our midsection—the center of metabolic activity in the body—as the solar plexus, which in Latin means "a gathering place for the sun." And in recognition of the supreme importance of metabolism, we have been taught to exert great effort to ensure its efficiency. Both metabolism and the sun benefit us most when we have just the right amount of each. Too much of either and we burn up or burn out.

Slowing Up

If you've chosen to read this book, you're likely doing so because you want to fire up your metabolism—you want more metabolic energy to lose weight, look lean, be healthier, and have more energy. Yet with all the latest diets, drugs, and weight-loss gizmos and gadgets, the majority of people fail to get what they want.

If you've worked for stronger metabolism but have not achieved success, there's one basic reason why: you're moving too fast.

The dizzying pace at which our culture propels itself is contrary to a happy and healthy life. We suffer from an avalanche of bodily ills and ailments of the soul that can be traced back to one simple cause: pace. I'm talking about the kind of speed that has us move unconsciously through our day, that pushes us beyond the body's natural capacity and leaves us unfulfilled and exhausted by day's end.

When moving through life too fast we inevitably eat fast, which destroys our metabolism and creates digestive upset. It results in meals eaten under a physiologic stress-response, which diminishes our calorie-burning power. It allows us little pleasure from food, decreasing cellular energy production and encouraging us to eat more. It shortens our breathing, which results in less oxygen intake and more fat accumulation. And it prompts us to abandon our deepest self and our true purpose for being here, leaving us with toxic thoughts and troublesome emotions that age the body and harden the heart.

Oddly enough, and despite our best intentions, we often attempt to remedy these ills by using strategies that make us feel worse. It's ironic how we mistakenly believe that diseases of speed can be cured by quick-fix methods. So we consume digestive aids and painkillers that yield debilitating side effects. We punish ourselves with excessive exercise for the crime of eating. We abuse ourselves with difficult diets and deny ourselves pleasure from food. And we avail ourselves of medical therapies that never truly address the reasons for our bodily breakdowns.

Maui taught us a great lesson. He harnessed the power of the sun not by speeding it up but by slowing it down. He aligned the sun with its natural course and pace and in doing so mastered a tremendous metabolic force.

Are you ready to master your own metabolic power with this same wisdom?

Fortunately, there's an effective remedy for this speed disease. It's called slowing down. We need to work less to achieve more. We need to stop fighting food and start embracing it. We need to stop punishing our bodies and start providing for them. We need to slow down and enjoy and then we'll get the results we've been looking for—and sooner than we expect.

The inescapable truth is that we can only achieve and sustain optimal metabolism when we eat, exercise, and live under an optimal emotional state. Our frame of mind directly impacts metabolism to such a degree that what we think and feel profoundly influences how we digest a meal. Metabolic power is not only about what you eat but who you are when you're eating. And it's not merely about how many calories you burn but how inspired you are about life.

Imagine, then, a relationship with food and your body that leaves you nourished and fulfilled each day. Imagine having the confidence to relax and enjoy the food you choose to eat. Imagine how good you'd feel if eating was a pure pleasure and exercise a delight. Imagine taking care of yourself with healthy, lifelong habits, not because you should do them but because they actually feel good. If you're ready to choose such a life, then you're ready to choose "slow."

The Slow Down Diet is about slowing down life to speed up metabolism. What I mean by "slowing down" is becoming more aware: Open. Centered. Present. Balanced. Create this experience for yourself and your mind, body, and breath will naturally align in a synergistic state. Immediate changes will occur in the nervous system, endocrine system, immune system, and the neuropeptide network throughout the body. The result is that you will burn calories at an optimal rate. You will digest and absorb nutrients at peak efficiency. You will circulate and combust oxygen for maximum energy release. Immunity will be enhanced. You'll step out of the stress-and-strain paradigm and into your own natural rhythm. The result is that you will feel more alive, energized, and abundant. Couple this with quality food choices and you'll begin to create the kind of metabolism that the wisdom of life has intended for you.

A New Way of Seeing Nutrition

As you ready yourself to work with food and metabolism in a whole new way, here are four of the most common nutrition myths you'll be leaving behind.

Myth #1: The best way to lose weight is to eat less and exercise more.

This formula intuitively sounds correct but is woefully incomplete. For the majority of people this approach fails over and over again. If it could work long-term it would have done so long ago. As you'll soon learn, underfeeding the body can slow metabolism, as can overexercising. Punishment gets you absolutely nowhere. True nourishment and joyous movement of the body will take you where you want to go.

Myth #2: The reason you eat too much is lack of willpower.
Fortunately, the experts are off the mark on this one too. As you'll discover, your willpower is better than you could have ever imagined. We overeat not because we're willpower weaklings but because we're physiologically driven to do so when our meals are deficient in relaxation, time, pleasure, awareness, and high-quality food.

Myth #3: As long as you eat the right foods in the right amounts, you'll ensure good health and lose weight.
This principle seems scientifically sound but it's caused way more damage than good. As you'll see, we can eat the healthiest food in the universe and in the perfect amount, but if we consume it in a state of anxious rushing, the physiologic stress-response will cause a dramatic rise in nutrient excretion and a deep decline in calorie-burning capacity. *What* you eat is only half the equation of good nutrition. *How* you eat is the other half.

Myth #4: The experts are your ultimate source of reliable and scientifically accurate nutrition information.
If only this were true. We experts certainly have our lofty place, but we love to disagree with one another and we constantly change our minds. In actual fact, the most definitive nutrition expertise is literally found inside you. It's called the enteric nervous system or ENS—the brain in the belly. This is your most faithful and accurate day-to-day dietary guide. The enteric nervous system has its own metabolic rules, which are *your* rules. This expert within you will help you choose which experts to follow outside you.

The principles you'll learn about in this book were born out of my lifelong exploration into food and healing. I've had the good fortune of diverse experience in the nutrition world. I was a featured lecturer and nutrition counselor for over ten years at a wonderful and world famous health resort, Canyon Ranch in the Berkshires. For over fifteen years I counseled and was a workshop leader and administrator at the Kripalu Center for Yoga and Health, one of the largest holistic health retreats in the country and another amazing laboratory for healing and transformation. I studied nutrition in college and graduate school, received my masters degree in psychology with an emphasis in eating psychology from Sonoma State University in California, did clinical training at Harvard in mind/body medicine, interned with numerous medical clinics and healers using leading edge nutritional therapeutics, assisted in nutrition-linked cancer research at the laboratories of Memorial Sloan-Kettering Cancer Center, and began a long career as a corporate consultant to food, vitamin, and health-related companies providing my expertise in product development, branding, communications, and corporate health, working in depth with notable organizations such as Johnson & Johnson and the Walt Disney Company. As a nutritional clinician I've worked successfully with children, the elderly, the rich and poor, the healthy and the diseased, prisoners, and athletes. I've counseled individuals challenged with biochemical disorders, eating disorders, and a great many people wanting to lose weight.

Oftentimes our work in the world is born out of our personal journey. From birth I was afflicted with severe asthma and allergies and nearly died on several occasions. I was shuffled from doctor to doctor but without relief. I couldn't run around like a normal child. I was desperate for health. At the age of five I heard a rumor that fruits and vegetables were good for you. Up until that time my diet was basically Cocoa Puffs for breakfast, Kool Aid and Marshmallow Fluff for lunch, and french fries and salami sandwiches for dinner. I asked my mother to buy apples and peas and carrots in a can because to my limited understanding, that's what fruits and vegetables were.

Miraculously, my health began to improve, and as my mother assisted me in incorporating other small changes in diet, my health flourished even more. So it was that from an early age I was able to make the profound connection that what went into my body had an effect on my health. In that era my father, who became a chiropractor in 1965, was learning about vitamins and homeopathy and bringing home lots of samples. Popping all those pills was one of the high points of my childhood—they catapulted me to the next level of wellness. I became convinced that good nutrition was the key to wellness and thus began my lifelong fascination with food, healing, personal transformation, and metabolism.

A New Definition of Metabolism

Many people use the word *metabolism* but few know what the word means. Indeed, if you asked a room filled with one hundred doctors and nutritionists "What is the definition of metabolism?" you would likely hear one hundred different answers. It's no surprise, then, that the average person would be confused about this topic.

Let's get down to basics and look at the classic textbook definition of *metabolism:* Metabolism is the sum total of all the chemical reactions in the body.

Are you surprised it's that simple? Of course, we can talk about the metabolism of such specific tissues as the liver and thyroid. We can talk about the metabolism of such specific substances as cholesterol. We can also talk about the metabolism of different body systems, such as digestive metabolism. People who say "I want to speed up my metabolism" are actually referring to calorie-burning metabolism, also known as thermic efficiency.

With this understanding, if we wanted to increase metabolism we'd make it our business to kick-start our body's chemical efficiency with exercise, drugs, the latest supplement, or a magic combination of foods. These approaches have certainly proved useful, but they are no longer adequate in describing metabolic reality.

This is so because metabolism doesn't occur in the body alone. It operates equally and simultaneously in body, mind, emotion, and spirit. Astounding research in the mind-body sciences has conclusively demonstrated the connection between what we think and feel and the chemistry of the body. Science has revealed the profound effects of the chemistries of stress, relaxation, pleasure, and depression, and the effects that even prayer, pets, and other people have on our lives.

Indeed, everything that happens in our world from birth until death is part and parcel of metabolism. All sensory input that impacts the human nervous system undergoes some form of digestion, assimilation, and elimination. In this very moment we're metabolizing elements of our last meal, words on this page, and important details of pivotal events that happened earlier this week or even previously in our lives. We metabolize our dreams, fears, and fantasies, our ups and downs, our jealousies and joys, the beauty that surrounds us, the betrayals we've suffered, and our fortunes and misfortunes—this in addition to all the frozen yogurt, chicken sandwiches, and sushi we eat. No wonder we take so many digestive aids.

Taking all these elements into consideration, our new definition of metabolism is this.

Metabolism is the sum total of all the chemical reactions in the body, plus the sum total of all our thoughts, feelings, beliefs, and experiences.

Not only is this definition more scientifically accurate and complete, you might also recognize it as intuitively correct. If you do, then you are in sync with such disciplines as Ayurveda and Chinese medicine, which for thousands of years have acknowledged the inseparable nature of mind, body, and cosmos. Chances are you've had many moments in which your metabolism was transformed by something other than food, drugs, or exercise. Can you recall a time when you were sitting at home feeling low energy and sorry for yourself, a time when if someone asked you "How's your metabolism?" you would have answered that it was sluggish and stuck? Then quite suddenly the phone rings and it's a love interest calling or it's someone calling you with good news about money. Your mood instantly skyrockets. You feel alive and optimistic. And in that moment, if someone asked again, "How's your metabolism?" you'd say it was humming.

So what happened? You had an enormous energy rush yet you didn't drink any coffee or take any drugs. It was a shift in your emotional world that ignited your body. That's how quickly metabolism can change.

In essence this book is about reclaiming metabolic power. It's about looking to see where we've given power away, leaked it out, and left ourselves with less. Many of us are accustomed to believing the erroneous notion that somehow we've been shortchanged on our metabolic allotment. We think we don't have enough to do what we need to do because somewhere the system has broken down. All we need to do is fix it with a vitamin, a drug, a diet, or an exercise program. If only we could find the right expert with the right answer, it would all work out.

The truth is, we are born metabolically powerful. If you've made it this far, the miraculous body you inhabit has done a worthy job. The forces of the universe launch us with a life-sustaining thrust that enables us to gather along our journey all that we need to continue to soar. But when we stay trapped in fight-or-flight survival physiology because of chronic, low-level stress; because of speed; because of a lack of breathing, awareness, and pleasure; and because of discordant rhythms and a negative personal story, we lose power big time. Furthermore, we lose power when we surrender our dignity and our inner authority to a job, to money, to the "experts," to hurtful emotions, and to a life of speed— to name just a few.

Reclaim your personal power in these areas and you reclaim a wealth of metabolic strength. It's as simple as that. And it's as profound as that. Personal power and metabolic power are one and the same.

Eight Universal Metabolizers

At the core of the Slow Down Diet are the eight universal metabolizers. I consider these to be some of the most important missing pieces in our collective metabolic puzzle, the next generation of powerful biologic rejuvenators that will prove themselves essential to our health at the deepest level of medical reality.

Despite existing for quite some time, the eight universal metabolizers have been long overlooked for several crucial reasons. First, we've been moving too fast to notice them, since their chemical power is activated only when the requisite level of "slowness" has been met. Second, we've believed that a metabolic enhancer must be exclusively of the order of a food, a pill, or a push-up, yet the eight universal metabolizers are of a different category. Let's call these metabolic enhancers *transubstantial,* meaning "above and beyond the realm of matter." You can't touch them, see them, bottle them, or sell them online, yet they are as fundamental to metabolism as vitamins, minerals, water, and exercise—perhaps even more so. Without them, we could never blossom into the vital and expressive creatures we are meant to be.

The eight universal metabolizers are:

- Relaxation
- Quality
- Awareness
- Rhythm

- Pleasure
- Thought
- Story
- The Sacred

As you'll see in the chapters to follow, each of these is a key that unlocks a door to a whole new means of transforming your nutritional metabolism, often in a manner that's quite unexpected and surprising in its ease. As a nutritional psychology expert I've seen far too many people frustrate themselves with low-calorie, low-fat, and low-life diets. I watched these same people exercise for months or years on end and still complain about sluggish metabolisms. Still others would lose weight using restrictive diets, yet they lived in a culinary prison that allowed no entry for pleasure and possibility of parole. Something more was clearly needed.

I found that mystery ingredient—the universal metabolizers—when I discovered yoga. While attending classes in breathing and body aware-ness, something remarkable happened. Quite unexpectedly, I had more energy and clarity than I'd ever had before. My digestion was suddenly stronger. I was visibly leaner, my craving for sweets disappeared, my appetite normalized, and I was aware of food and of enjoying it in a whole new way—all this from breathing in more oxygen and practicing more attention. I didn't adopt a self-punishing system, I didn't work obsessively hard, and I didn't fight food.

As I incorporated simple yoga-based breathing and body awareness techniques into my consulting practice, nutritional breakthroughs occurred for my clients. I was amazed how those with chronic complaints saw fast progress and relief. Many digestive problems cleared in days when clients learned the techniques of stress-free eating. Weight loss finally came for those who embraced the sacred, tuned in to their gut wisdom—the messages from the enteric nervous system—and allowed themselves more pleasure. Still others said good-bye to binge eating and overeating, improving their energy level and mental acuity and discovering a new relationship with food.

The bottom line was this: These folks achieved more by doing less. The people I'm speaking of stopped fighting food and started embracing it. They stopped denying and began nourishing themselves. They relaxed when they ate and so increased their metabolism. They chose healthy pleasure over pain. They worked with natural rhythms rather than against them. They ceased being victimized by food, by their bodies, and by anyone else's standards and instead took responsibility for making simple but profound changes that created an empowered metabolic state. They slowed down and trusted life.

I've had the great satisfaction of witnessing many metabolic transformations in my work at Canyon Ranch and at the Kripalu Center, with corporate clients, in live workshops with thousands of students, and in our work at the Institute of the Psychology of Eating, which has reached literally hundreds of thousands of people around the world. Surprisingly, these changes are quite commonplace and are available to anyone.

A Slow Down Success Story

Sandy dieted for six years without lasting results. She'd go from one system to the next, but any amount of weight she lost would quickly find its way back on. She complained of ongoing gastric reflux—heartburn—and bouts of overeating. She lived in a relentless battle with food that consumed a significant chunk of her life energy. Despite a clean bill of health from her doctors, Sandy was convinced that her problem was a sluggish metabolism. She was tired of struggling with food and exercise but didn't know which way to turn.

In less than six weeks' time working together, Sandy lost fifteen pounds and within four months she was a total of forty-five pounds lighter while eating more fat and exercising less. Her war with food was over, and she finally had what she wanted. Here's what we did.

First, we focused on quality. When we met, Sandy's diet consisted of very little fresh or homemade food. She ate lots of artificially sweetened and mass-produced products with poor-quality fat; she ate almost no low-toxic, nutrient-dense foods. Using the guidelines you'll read about in chapter 2, we improved the quality of Sandy's diet. In doing so, the quantity of food she ate naturally began to diminish. When the body fails to receive the quality nutrition it desires, it isn't always smart enough to call for better food—it screams "more food!"

Next, we looked at rhythm. Sandy had been skipping breakfast, eating a small and hurried lunch, and having a big dinner after work sometime around eight o'clock. Like Sandy, what most people don't realize is that the body metabolizes food most effectively at midday, specifically at the point when the sun is highest in the sky. Research shows that we burn calories best at lunch. Late evening and early morning hours are the least efficient times for metabolizing food. Sumo wrestlers don't gain weight by eating tons of Ben & Jerry's ice cream; they eat the same rice, vegetables, and sushi as their fellow countrymen. The difference is that they eat this food in great quantity and late at night.

Sandy didn't realize that she was on the Sumo diet. I recommended that she eat a real breakfast, a good-sized lunch, and a small dinner. She would be eating more calories but concentrating them at the time of peak metabolic efficiency. And by taking more time to eat, she would be literally mixing more oxygen with her meal, resulting in greater calorie-burning capacity and more robust digestion.

Next, because Sandy described herself as a fast eater, I asked her to relax and breathe. There's something scientists call the cephalic phase digestive response (CPDR). *Cephalic* means "of the head." The cephalic phase digestive response is a fancy term for the body's experience of the taste, aroma, satisfaction, visuals, and overall pleasure of a meal. Depending upon which research study you consider, anywhere from 20 to 80 percent of our calorie-burning power, digestive power, and assimilation of

specific nutrients comes directly from CPDR—the "head phase" of digestion. By rushing through her meals Sandy significantly diminished her
metabolism. Her rapid-fire eating was locking her body into a stress
response, which dramatically decreases digestion and calorie-burning ability. After incorporating simple deep-breathing exercises, the increased
oxygenation and blood flow to her digestive system stimulated thermic
efficiency—her calorie-burning power. Breathing and relaxation also
reversed her stress-induced digestive shutdown, which completely cleared
her chronic gastric reflux.

After these successes, I asked Sandy to do something that initially
seemed beyond reason. I suggested she enjoy eating and allow herself to
feel nourished and to let go of any guilt no matter what she ate. This
was especially difficult for Sandy because she had spent much of her
adult life fighting food. For the first time ever, Sandy was truly considering the possibility of not inflicting pain upon herself but inflicting
pleasure instead. Indeed, pleasure is a powerful metabolizer that
increases oxygenation and blood flow and decreases the production of
cortisol and insulin, ultimately helping to burn fat and build muscle. It
also induces parasympathetic nervous system dominance, which activates full digestive metabolism and calorie-burning power.

Finally, we dealt with Sandy's biggest challenge—overeating. To her
surprise, I explained that she had never been able to conquer her overeating problem for one simple reason: the problem didn't actually exist.
In my experience, I've learned that about nine out of ten people who
claim to be overeaters really have a different issue—they don't eat when
they eat. Because of a deficiency of a key universal metabolizer—
awareness—many of us doze off while we eat. Failing to notice our food,
we completely bypass the body's satiation mechanism. The result is that
we hunger for more.

As you may recall from junior high school biology class, all organisms on the planet—be they amoeba, lizard, lion, or human being—are
programmed for two things in common: to seek pleasure and to avoid
pain. When we eat, we are pursuing the pleasure of food and avoiding
the pain of hunger. If we fail to pay attention to the food, the brain

interprets this missed experience as hunger and signals us to eat more. We mistakenly think our problem is one of willpower when instead we simply need to be more present when we eat.

The net result of Sandy's work was, for her, astounding. She catalyzed a permanent change in weight and felt energized with food for the first time since her teen years. Slowing down and working with the wisdom of the body enabled her to increase her metabolic speed.

Are you beginning to see the possibilities for your own metabolic breakthrough?

Each of the eight universal metabolizers that I've listed above is discussed in its own chapter here in this book. Each chapter represents one week of the eight-week Slow Down program. Every chapter begins with insights and research, findings that help you become familiar with the principles of that week's metabolic enhancer, and ends with practical tools and techniques that will help you focus your attention on implementing those principles. You'll become like a personal client of mine and experience benefits that are immediate, lasting, and rewarding.

The eight-week Slow Down program lays the foundation for something special to happen in your metabolic world. For as you empower yourself to explore your unique relationship to food, to let go of fear and guilt, and to be with your body in a dignified and loving way, you likewise empower your metabolism. The chemistry of the body is that simple, and that elegant. Make this program fun, see it as an exploration, become ever more interested in your own nutritional nuances, and your success is assured. Keep a journal and write down your activities and reflections at the end of each day. Record what you ate and how you felt afterward. Note your insights, focus on the positive, and acknowledge your progress, no matter how small the step or significant the leap.

Are you ready to let go of the habits that don't work and claim as yours the ones that do? Are you prepared to embrace the full range of richly abundant metabolic enhancers that can ignite both body and soul? Because science has focused on a narrow view of what health can really be, our fitness experts are satisfied when we've burned enough calories or reached our target heart rate. Our dietary gurus are happy when our milk has enough vitamin D and our juice has enough vitamin C. Little have we realized that our diet has been collectively deficient in some important nutrients that have been around for quite some time, yet were somehow overlooked: vitamin L—love, vitamin H—happiness, and vitamin S—soul. You won't find these essential nutrients listed on the side panel of your cereal box, but don't let that absence fool you. If something is truly nourishing for the soul then it is literally nourishing for the body. And that nourishment is what fuels metabolism.

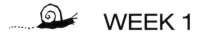 WEEK 1

The Metabolic Power of Relaxation

If time, so fleeting, must see humans die,
let it be filled with good food and good talk,
and then embalmed with the perfumes
of conviviality.

M. F. K. FISHER

Gandhi once said, "There is more to life than increasing its speed." But you'd never know it by the way many of us eat. Eating under stress is not only commonplace, it's socially acceptable and often a prerequisite for managing a job, maintaining a family, or having a life. Eva, an office worker, tells an all-too-typical story.

"I'm always overloaded with work, so food has to fit into my work schedule, which means nibbling at my desk whenever I can. I usually eat two meals a day at the office, but they're not real meals. I work, nibble, answer the phone, nibble, type, nibble, run around the office, nibble. I know I need to eat slower, but with my schedule I could never manage it."

If you're a fast and furious eater, it's time to change gears. That's because the slower you eat, the faster you metabolize.

Can you recall what your body sensations are when you eat during a state of anxiety or stress? Most people report such symptoms as heartburn, cramping, gas, digestive pains, belching, and intense hunger. During stress the body automatically shifts into the classic fight-or-flight response. This feature of the central nervous system evolved over millions of years into a brilliant safety mechanism that supports us during life-threatening events—confronting hostile attackers, experiencing natural disasters, quickly evading or forcibly overcoming anyone or anything.

In the moment the stress response is activated, heart rate speeds up, blood pressure increases, respiration quickens, hormones that help provide immediate energy such as adrenaline, noradrenaline, and cortisol are released into the circulatory system, blood flow is rerouted away from the midsection and toward the head for quick thinking and to the arms and legs for the power necessary to fight or flee. Most importantly, in a full-blown stress response, the digestive system completely shuts down. It makes perfect sense that when you're fending off an angry gorilla, you don't need to waste energy digesting your Froot Loops. All the body's metabolic functions must be geared directly for survival.

So picture yourself anxiously rushing from your apartment to the office while munching on a muffin, or grabbing a fast lunch while you're overloaded with work and thinking about everything but food, or eating a meal when you're upset because the universe is being uncooperative about conforming to your humble demands. During these moments the body hasn't a clue that what you're experiencing is not life threatening, because it is genetically programmed to initiate the fight-or-flight response the instant the brain perceives stress. This means that, depending on the intensity of the stress you're experiencing, each of the physiological changes that characterize the fight-or-flight response is activated, including some degree of digestive shutdown.

So if you've ever eaten in an anxious state and had the feeling afterward that food is just sitting in your stomach, that's exactly what it's doing. It's waiting between several minutes and several hours for the body to kick back into normal digestive functioning.

The famous capitalist Malcolm Forbes once remarked in defense of fast foods that, "Just because you can get it in a hurry doesn't mean it's junk." Perhaps this is true. But what he didn't recognize in that statement is that just because you eat something in a hurry doesn't mean your body will assimilate it any faster. You can eat the healthiest meal in the solar system, but if you eat it in an anxious state, your digestion is dramatically diminished—your mood has affected your food. Salivary enzyme content in the mouth is reduced, the breakdown of protein, fat, and carbohydrate macromolecules in the stomach is impaired, and blood flow to the small intestines is decreased as much as fourfold, which translates into decreased assimilation of vitamins, minerals, and other nutrients. It's not only important what we eat, then, but the mental state we are in when we eat.

The Stress—Metabolism Connection

The key to understanding the profound link between metabolism and stress is the central nervous system (CNS). The portion of the CNS that exerts the greatest influence on gastrointestinal function is called the autonomic nervous system (ANS); this aspect of the nervous system is responsible for getting your stomach churning, getting the enzymatic secretions in the digestive process flowing, and keeping the dynamic process of nutrient absorption into the bloodstream on the move. The ANS also tells your body when not to be in digesting mode, such as when there's no food in your belly or when you're in fight-or-flight response.

Two subdivisions of the ANS help it accomplish its dual task of digestive arousal and digestive inhibition: the sympathetic and parasympathetic branches. The sympathetic branch activates the stress response and suppresses digestive activity. The parasympathetic branch relaxes the body and activates digestion. It might be helpful to think of these two parts of the nervous system as on-and-off switches.

| When parasympathetic nervous system active | DIGESTION ON | Stress response off: body relaxed |
| When sympathetic nervous system active | DIGESTION OFF | Stress response on: body in fight-or-flight mode |

Simply put, the same part of our brain that turns on stress turns off digestion. And conversely, the part of the brain that turns on the relaxation response turns on full, healthy digestive power. Eating healthy food is only half of the story of good nutrition. Being in the ideal state to digest and assimilate food is the other half.

Chen, a charismatic forty-six-year-old doctor of Chinese medicine, was plagued by nagging digestive upset despite overall great health and a vast knowledge of natural healing. He felt that maybe it was time to look at his diet and requested my help. When I asked some basic questions about his eating habits, I was quite surprised at the answers. Chen would stop at McDonalds on his way to work and eat two Egg McMuffins for breakfast in the car while rushing through city traffic. For lunch he'd zip to the same McDonalds and eat two Big Macs in the car as he drove back to the office. After work, he ate two slices of pizza. Chen informed me that he wanted to feel better but he wasn't willing to cook, bring a lunch to work, eat vegetables, or give up McDonalds. Go figure.

I told him I suspected I could actually help him despite the impossible limitations he was giving me to work with. Here is the simple strategy to which Chen reluctantly agreed. He had to eat his Big Macs while the car was parked and take twenty minutes to enjoy them slowly and sensually. He had to do the same with his Egg McMuffins at breakfast. He needed to take time to slow down with food, and with life. He needed to breathe deeply before, during, and after his meals.

Two weeks later Chen called me in an excited state with some wonderful news to tell. First, his digestive symptoms had disappeared. And then he said, "You won't believe this, really, but I *hate* Big Macs.

The Biochemical Burden of Stress[1]

Consider the facts in the following chart to help inspire you to experience the joys of slow, relaxed, and civilized eating.

The stress response will cause:

↓ **Nutrient absorption**—primarily due to decreased oxygenation and gastrointestinal blood flow; decreased enzymatic production in stomach, pancreas, and liver; decreased bile flow from gall bladder.

↑ **Nutrient excretion**—urinary loss of calcium, magnesium, potassium, zinc, chromium, selenium, and various microminerals.

↑ **Nutrient deficiencies**—particularly vitamin C, vitamin B, iron, zinc, selenium.

↑ **Blood cholesterol**—stress by itself will raise LDL levels.

↑ **Serum triglycerides**—instantly increases during stress response.

↑ **Blood platelet aggregation**—a major risk factor in heart disease.

↑ **Salt retention**—can lead to high blood pressure.

↑ **Cortisol**—associated with weight gain, abdominal obesity, and inability to lose weight or build muscle. Excessive output prematurely ages the body.

↓ **Gut flora populations**—healthy intestinal bacteria are destroyed by stress. This can lead to immune problems, skin disorders, nutrient deficiencies, and digestive distress.

↓ **Oxygen supply**—influences all aspects of metabolism.

↓ **Thermic efficiency**—your ability to burn calories is diminished.

↑ **Hydrochloric acid production**—increases probability of ulcers.

↓ **Growth hormone**—a key hormone in growing, healing, and rebuilding body tissues. Helps to burn fat and build muscle.

↓ **Salivary secretions**—decreased digestion of starches and decreased oral immune factors.

↓ **Thyroid hormone**—can lead to a decrease in metabolic activity throughout the body.

↑ **Swallowing rate**—a fast swallowing rate is a likely factor in digestive upset.

↓ **Gastric emptying time**—can lead to diarrhea and larger food particles prematurely entering small intestines, a probable factor in food allergies, sensitivities, and various disease conditions.

↑ **Gastric emptying time**—can lead to constipation. Also a risk factor in diseases of the colon.

↑ **Food sensitivities and allergies**—plenty of anecdotal evidence, most likely due to decreased immunity and leaky gut.

↑ **Erratic function of LES**—lower esophageal sphincter opens inappropriately, causing gastric reflux (also known as heartburn).

↑ **Insulin resistance**—chronic low-level stress may cause target cells to become unresponsive to insulin, a factor in diabetes, weight gain, heart disease, and aging.

↓ **Eicosanoids**—this important class of master hormones includes prostaglandins, thromboxanes, leukotrienes. Influences energy level and numerous metabolic functions.

↑ **Risk of osteoporosis**—bone density has been shown to decrease in stressed and depressed women. Stress increases urinary excretion, of calcium, magnesium, and boron.

↑ **Oxidative stress**—prematurely ages the body. A precursor to numerous diseases.

↓ **Muscle mass**—means more flab and a slower metabolism.

↓ **Sex hormones**—can mean lower sex drive, low energy, decreased muscle mass.

↑ **Inflammation**—the basis of many significant ailments, including brain and heart disease.

↓ **Mitochondria**—these are the energy powerhouses of the cell. When the sheer number of these tiny cellular organelles are diminished, we literally produce less energy. Can lead to chronic fatigue.

↓ **Kidney function**—means toxicity, electrolyte imbalance, water retention, heart disease.

I've been eating them for fifteen years and I can't stand them. Have you ever tried to savor a Big Mac? You can't. You have to eat it fast and smother it with lots of ketchup to hide the taste."

Chen was not a relaxed eater. He had plenty of patients to see throughout the day and seemingly little time for self-nourishment. The simple act of taking time to slow down and eat shifted him from sympathetic to parasympathetic dominance, and his digestive upset quickly disappeared. When this happened, his body wisdom was finally able to give feedback about his food choices, and he subsequently gave up Big Macs naturally and effortlessly. He didn't need to use his willpower to resist a favorite food or exert mental force to make better choices. All he did was savor a Big Mac.

Are you beginning to understand the metabolic power of relaxation? Can you see how eating in the natural and necessary state of parasympathetic dominance can yield breakthroughs with food and metabolism?

Lessons from the French

One of the more fascinating examples I know of that illustrates the profound difference between relaxed and rushed eating comes from European culture. Have you ever been to France? Do you know how the French "do it" when it comes to food? When asked this question most people who are familiar with the culture comment that the French take a few hours for lunch, they drink a generous amount of red wine with their meals, they eat lots of cheese and high-fat foods, their portions tend to be smaller, their midday meal is the largest of the day, they're fanatic about using fresh foods and high-quality ingredients, they don't exercise as much as Americans, they smoke a lot, they're thinner, and they dine and celebrate their meals as opposed to eating and running. Until recently, the French didn't even have a term for "fast food."

Compare this to Americans, many of whom often take only several minutes for breakfast and lunch as opposed to an hour or more; who take their largest meal of the day at dinner rather than at lunch; who don't, on the whole, drink wine with meals, insist on high-quality ingredients, and make each meal a cultural celebration to remember. Americans also eat larger portions, are more apt to exercise, and have larger bodies.

In the 1990s, researchers began comparing health in America and health in France and they came up with some eye-opening news. What they discovered was that the French consume a significantly higher percentage of dietary fat per capita than Americans. Man for man and woman for woman, the French eat a lot more fat throughout the year. This means that they should have higher blood cholesterol levels and a higher rate of heart disease, but as it turns out these rates for the French are significantly lower than for Americans. This was as earthshaking a revelation to the scientific community as a UFO landing because heart disease and blood cholesterol are supposed to increase as people eat more fat, not go the other way.

We put our best medical minds to work on this dilemma and looked at as many explanations as we could. Scientists reasoned that there was a mystery ingredient in the French diet that gives them their healthy edge—they surmised it to be red wine. Then they isolated the active chemical components of the red wine—polyphenols. This was the supposed X-factor exerting a heart-protective effect on the French.

Days later the front page of major newspapers across the country told us "Drink more wine." This, of course, caused a major stir because it contradicted so many other studies that told us how alcohol kills brain cells, suppresses the immune system, damages the liver, mutates fetuses, and otherwise wreaks havoc on society through inebriation and addiction. Who to believe?

Our solution to this controversy was to isolate the polyphenols out of the wine, encapsulate them, bottle them, and sell them in health food stores across the land. The problem solved, researchers could now sleep soundly knowing that little red-wine polyphenols pills are all that stand between Americans and the heart-healthy French.

But let's take a closer look. None of the researchers on this project really considered the big picture. First and foremost, the French consistently eat under parasympathetic dominance—the physiological state of relaxation and maximum digestive function. Even if they are stressed out, taking a generous amount of time to eat a meal, savoring it, and schmoozing with other Frenchmen and Frenchwomen probably helps them let go. And if that doesn't ease their tensions, then the red wine certainly will.

Though the fast-food culture is gradually taking hold, the French (and other Europeans) on the whole aren't doing power lunches like we practice in America. The context for their eating isn't business. It's pleasure. As a culture they place a high value not only on food but on nourishment. Eating isn't considered to be some nuisance biological requirement to get out of the way. They take time during the day to relax, celebrate, and acknowledge the deep human need to dine. It's not the polyphenols in the red wine that keep their cholesterol level and heart disease in check. It's their parasympathetic nervous system. It's the optimum state of digestion and assimilation that they consistently eat under as a result of their frame of mind.

A stressed eater = sympathetic dominance = digestive shutdown

A relaxed eater = parasympathetic dominance = full digestive force

---

Here's one last lesson from the French. An American geologist I know was sent to France to supervise a three-week dig in the countryside. Because the time allotted for completing the job was too short, she was quickly frustrated when at noontime each day her French crew would disappear into town for a two-and-a-half hour lunch. After a week she explained to the men that the company had put them on a very tight schedule and they needed to eat lunch on site. They discussed it among themselves and cheerfully agreed.

The next day the crew brought in a mysterious truck that sat all morning in the parking area. When lunchtime arrived, they opened the truck and out came tables, tablecloths, silverware, china, flowers, a portable kitchen, and a lavish supply of food. They dined for two and a half hours amid rocks and rubble, enjoyed their wine, and were genuinely pleased with themselves to have fulfilled the American boss's request to eat at work.

Relax and Burn Calories

Have you ever had the experience where you've gone on vacation, eaten much more than usual, and lost weight? About one out of five people I've polled answered this question in the affirmative. Others will say they ate significantly more food yet maintained the same weight. According to the old paradigm of nutrition, this is impossible at best (or else it is a miracle). But to our new understanding about digestion and metabolism, the reason for this weight loss is simple to understand. While on vacation many of us do something that is highly unusual for us. We relax. We move from chronic sympathetic dominance to a parasympathetic state. Our frame of mind changes our metabolism to such a degree that we can eat more and yet lose weight.

Yvonne, a graduate student, told this story. "I went to Italy for a semester and really let myself go with food. I got off my diet and lived it up. I ate bread, cheese, desserts, gelato, creamy everything, and lots of pasta. I could hardly believe it, but I lost eight pounds while I was there."

Arthur, a contractor, had this to say. "I went to a resort in Jamaica for a couple of weeks. I was exhausted from a job and I deserved a break. I ate a lot, drank a lot, slept on the beach, and I think I might have taken a walk. My wife still talks about how I lost seven pounds on the 'hedonist diet.'"

Ella works on a sailing ship half the year on Nantucket and the other half in the Virgin Islands. She noticed that whenever she arrived in the Virgin Islands she'd lose around fifteen pounds within a month, without any change in diet or exercise. Can you guess what made the difference? Not only did she love the Virgin Islands more than Nantucket, she also realized that she felt more attractive on the islands. "The men native to the Virgin Islands don't care how big you are. They actually prefer large women. On Nantucket I don't get much attention from men. When I get to the islands, the men think I'm hot. I never worry about calories there, and I eat whatever I want and enjoy it. I'm a completely different person and my metabolism totally changes."

The point, of course, is not to reach for absolutely everything you want to eat or to take more vacations in the Virgin Islands. The point is that many of us need to let go and live because we'll relax more and metabolize better.

The scientifically documented connection between weight gain and stress is rather compelling. Numerous clinical studies have shown that conditions with high cortisol production are strongly associated with fat accumulation.[2] That's because one of cortisol's chemical responsibilities is to signal the body to store fat and not build muscle.

The Gift of Time

During week 1, you can help yourself slow down and relax and hence increase your nutritional metabolism with this one simple exercise: Commit to providing yourself the gift of more time at each meal. Trust that the world can wait while you take a few more minutes with your food and reclaim your right to dine.

- If you eat breakfast in five minutes, bump it up to ten. If you normally take ten minutes, increase it to fifteen or twenty.

- Give yourself at least thirty minutes for lunch and dinner. See if you can increase it to an hour.

- Rearrange your home and work schedules as best as you can to provide yourself with more time. Honestly look to see where you can find these extra moments.

- As best as you can, enroll your family, co-workers, and boss in creating more time and relaxation with meals. Find a "slow down buddy" and support each other in dining.

- Eat only in the sitting position. Choose to not answer the cell phone, home phone, work phone, pager, e-mails, or to engage in any form of work while you dine.

Recall that cortisol is the key hormone released in significant quantities during acute and chronic stress. Rats and monkeys experimentally subjected to stress will initially show elevated cortisol levels followed by weight gain. This occurs despite the fact that they're eating a normal amount of food. Indeed, many people complain that even though they're eating a lower-calorie diet and exercising more, they still can't lose weight. More often than not, stress is the reason. This is especially the case for those who experience weight gain around the midsection, as excess cortisol production has the strange effect of fattening up the belly.

So if you're the kind of person who seems to be doing everything right for weight loss but are stuck on the same plateau, ask yourself about stress. Do you live a hurried life? Are you eating at warp speed? Does your job require that you live in a state of fight or flight? If so, then no amount of calorie counting or treadmilling will get you where you want to go. Your task is to do something of the greatest possible difficulty. Relax. Stop producing so much cortisol. Take a deep breath into your life, be a little more peaceful, and give your calories a chance to burn.

Chronic stress can also increase the output of insulin, another hormone strongly associated with weight gain. The pancreas produces insulin whenever there is a rapid rise in blood sugar. One of the ways that insulin lowers blood glucose is by telling the body to aggressively store excess dietary carbohydrates as fat. Insulin also signals the body not to release any stored fat. Chronic stress and its attendant insulin output is especially problematic in a condition known as insulin resistance, in which blood-sugar levels remain elevated despite increased insulin output due to an unresponsiveness of target cells for this hormone. Couple this with the typical high-carbohydrate snacks we consume when feeling anxious and unloved and we pave the way for quick and easy weight gain. When it comes to weight loss, then, it is as important to relax and count our blessings as it is to count our calories.

So imagine yourself worrying about your weight, following a

forced and flaccid diet, and convinced of your unworthiness to exist if you can't shrink your body down to some perfect size. These self-perpetuated messages will literally put you in a state of chronic low-level stress. Though you're consuming less calories by dieting, you're producing more cortisol and insulin, which is signaling your body to gain weight. In medical terms, chronic stress decreases thermic efficiency—your ability to burn calories and metabolize stored fat.

The bottom line is this.

Worrying about fat increases fat. Anxiety about weight loss causes your body to put fat on and retain it.

Many people use anxiety and stress to motivate themselves to lose weight. For example, "If I don't lose eight pounds for the party, I won't go," or "I'll never look good until I lose weight." This self-chosen stress feels energizing because it produces such alertness hormones as adrenaline and noradrenaline; over time though, these fight-or-flight hormones can diminish metabolism.

Even though I've seen many extraordinary examples over the years, it still seems like magic when people share their stories of how relaxation transformed their bodies. Terry, a fifty-five-year-old schoolteacher, lost nine pounds in four weeks without changing anything in her diet. She simply decided to stop worrying about everything she ate. Jody, a thirty-one-year-old writer, lost five pounds in a week—the same "last five pounds" she was trying to take off for years—when she finally decided to stop obsessing about five silly pounds. Esther, age forty-eight, was a long-term dieter who never really lost anything. After several months on a "no-diet" diet without any guilt or self-imposed rules she still didn't lose anything—except guilt, fear, and dietary misery.

The point is this: you don't need to worry any more or punish yourself about food. It is totally counterproductive to stress yourself out about weight loss because that same stress causes you to put weight on.

Relax and Build Bones

We all know calcium supplements can help build bones, but have you heard of the bone-building power of inner peace? Research has shown an unmistakable effect of stress on bone density. Mice exposed to a three-week period of living in overcrowded cages showed significant bone demineralization—loss of calcium, phosphorous, magnesium, and iron.[3] (City dwellers take note.) They also showed significant losses in micro-mineral concentrations associated with bone health—zinc, boron, chromium, and cobalt.

The glucocorticoids, a class of stress hormones that includes cortisol, are largely responsible for the bone-wasting effects of stress. These hormones actually block the assimilation of calcium in the intestines and severely restrict the amount of calcium available for bone growth. Excessive secretion of glucocorticoids, as seen in chronic stress, will cause urinary calcium loss, interfere with the growth and division of specialized precursor cells in the ends of your bones, and will even increase the rate at which bone tissue is broken down. These bone-crushing effects of stress have been most clearly observed experimentally in female monkeys subject to everyday stresses. We also see it in people with Cushing's syndrome (a disease in which cortisol is hypersecreted), and in patients who are treated with massive doses of glucocorticoids for a disease condition.

So if you think that a calcium supplement is all you need to protect against your bones skipping out on you, think again. America has one of the highest rates of calcium intake in the world and still has one of the highest rates of osteoporosis. Something's wrong with this picture. The successful equation for bone density is not about getting more calcium. It's about excreting less. We literally lose calcium in the urine within minutes of feeling stress; this is the same calcium that moments before was in your bones. One study conducted by the National Institutes of Health and published in the *New England Journal of Medicine* confirmed that past or current depression in women is strongly associated with bone loss. Depressed females had bone density measurements as much as 13 percent lower than nondepressed subjects. This study conclusively demonstrated that bone health and mental health go hand in hand.[4]

It's instructive to note that stress isn't the only factor that would cause us to excrete urinary calcium. Other calcium excretors include caffeine, alcohol, air pollution, cigarette smoke, excess sugar, excess animal protein, and phosphoric acid (found in many cola-flavored sodas).[5] Wrap these all up into the typical office-worker lifestyle and we're pissing away a most precious mineral at an alarming rate. So if you've been bombarded with the message to "take more calcium," it's time to look at the big picture.

A woman who attended one of my workshops approached me afterward anxious to tell me her story. Despite a lifetime of exercise, a healthy high-calcium diet, and no family history of the disease, Arlene had recently been diagnosed with osteoporosis at age forty-two. Her doctors were stumped and she was devastated by her diagnosis because it didn't seem to make sense. Upon hearing me mention the connection between stress and bone loss, Arlene had a personal revelation. Her job had made her sick. She had been working at an intensely high-stress, high-demand publishing job for over sixteen years and it consumed most of her life. For the first time she realized she could make a change to a more satisfying job, a change that could be as important as taking her medication.

True to her word, Arlene soon left her job with the publisher she'd been with for most of her career. She found a magazine that offered a more sane working environment, a healthier schedule, and a real lunch break. She still had her share of job stress, but she also had more nourishing relationships with her co-workers and some precious moments of relaxation during her day. When we spoke over a year later, Arlene had this story to tell.

"I always accepted a high-stress work life because I didn't think I had a choice. At some point it just became normal. I've been fanatic over the years about diet and exercise, but I see now that I chronically ate under stress, and I know it took its toll on me. . . . I'm happy at work now for the first time ever, and I make sure to eat when I'm relaxed. . . . The proof that it's all working is I've reversed my osteoporosis when no other approach was succeeding. I know it's more than the calcium. It's me." When Arlene first had her "aha" experience about stress and bone disease she did something she hadn't done enough of before—she tuned in to her body wisdom and let her inner knowing speak. She gave herself the luxury of believing she had a choice and a voice in the world she created for herself.

Can you see the amazing metabolic changes we can make by empowering ourselves in all our life choices, large and small? Do you understand how bone health depends not only on the calcium in your food but on the feelings in your heart and the thoughts in your head? Bones need more than nutrition. They need to be nourished.

Of course, stress is a normal part of living and serves a healthy function. However, the physiologic stress-response was designed to function for only minutes at a time and in life-threatening situations. In fact, in the first few minutes of a full-on stress response our metabolism reaches its peak efficiency. When the response is prolonged, day after day, that's when the very survival tool that's supposed to save us begins to tear us down.

Week 1: Your Primary Task

Would you describe yourself as a fast eater, a moderate eater, or a slow eater? If you answered "slow," congratulations. If not, this is your primary task for week 1 and well beyond: transform yourself into a slow eater. Any time you eat with others, secretly hold a contest. You win if you finish the meal last!

Week 1 is your opportunity to graduate from the habit of high-speed eating and elevate your body to parasympathetic dominance during meals—the optimal state of digestion, assimilation, and calorie burning. It's a time to imprint in your consciousness now and forevermore that fast food is out and "slow food" is in. It's your new lifestyle. If you've tried different diets and nutritional systems but haven't been able to consistently stay with one approach, then it's time to change your strategy. Let's put first things first. Rather than focus on *what* to eat, it's time to get clear about *how* to eat.

Exercise: Lifestyle Inventory

During week 1 of the Slow Down Diet, eat your usual fare. But now just relax and slow down like never before. Let go of the need to know "the right things to eat." We'll look at that dietary issue more closely in weeks 2 and 3.

For now, find a suitable and special journal that you can use for the exercises and activities you'll be doing throughout this book. Then, take a moment to consider your own stress-free or stress-full eating styles by answering some of the following questions.

- Do you tend to eat more when feeling anxious? Or do you eat less at those times? Might you do one or the other depending on the situation?
- What kinds of circumstances prompt you to eat this way: particular times of the day? certain settings? specific days of the week? Is anxious eating work-related for you? Is it family-related?
- Approximately how often do you eat under stress? Can you express this in a percentage of your total eating time? (As an example, some people eat under stress only 5 percent of the time, some 85 percent of the time.)
- Do you tend to eat certain foods when feeling stressed out? List as many of those foods as you can. Which ones do you eat the most?
- Do you feel full after stressful eating or do you feel hungry? Are there any common physical symptoms you've noticed during or after such times?
- How much time do you take for your repast during stressful eating episodes? Do you taste your food? Do you chew it much or do you shovel it down?

Next, think of the meals when you're relaxed, enjoying yourself and your food, perhaps in good company, when you're satisfied with what you have and fulfilled once your meal is complete. How often does this occur for you? What percentage of the time? Do you eat any particular foods during relaxed meals? How much time do you take? Where do you eat these meals? With whom? When? How do you feel after a stress-free meal? What are the sensations in your body?

Vitamin T—time for meals—is a most fundamental nutritional requirement and one that is lacking in the diets of many of us in the "civilized" world. By including more time with food you can elevate yourself from a mammal that feeds to a human being who eats. The result is that you'll nourish yourself with food rather than chaotically shovel nutrients into your digestive tract. And in doing so, your metabolism will be maximized.

Even if you feel pressed for time, the good news is that it takes less than a minute to de-stress the body and move it into maximum nutritional metabolism. Fortunately, you needn't sell your home and move to France to achieve this. You can eat stress-free anywhere and anytime and experience the rewards almost instantly.

The royal road to shortcut the physiologic stress-response and bring you to relaxed, slow eating is conscious breathing.

Here's why.

Every emotional state has a corresponding brain-wave frequency and breath pattern. Picture yourself driving through an intersection and slamming on the brakes because someone runs a red light. If you could notice your breathing pattern, in that moment of a near-death experience, you'd witness yourself holding your breath. Think about it. The breathing pattern of stress and anxiety is shallow, arrhythmic, and infrequent. Once you realize the accident didn't happen and your life is spared, you'd likely exhale with a deep sigh. The body's natural intelligence automatically deep breathes us the moment it realizes a life-threatening circumstance has passed.

When we are in a stressful state, if we consciously adopt the deep and rhythmic breathing pattern characteristic of the *relaxed* state we fool the central nervous system. The brain says something like, "Hey, I thought I was a nervous wreck but I'm breathing like a relaxed person. I must be relaxed!" A signal is sent from the frontal cortex of the brain (the thinking center), to the spinal nerves, to target organs throughout the body. The endocrine system is brought in as well to deactivate the stress response. The result is a shift from a state of low digestive activity to full digestive force.

I've watched many people cure or dramatically curtail the symptoms of irritable bowel syndrome, heartburn, constipation, chronic gastric upset, fatigue after meals, and a host of digestive complaints by regularly using the two simple breathing techniques that follow.

Exercise: Check In and Breathe

At every meal or snack, and any time food is about to pass across your lips, ask yourself "Am I about to eat under stress? Is my mind in high gear?" If the answer is yes, pause. Then take ten long, slow, deep breaths. Ideally, your deep-breathing experience would follow this sequence:

Sit in a comfortable position with spine straight, feet flat on the floor.

Eyes can be open or closed.

Deeply inhale, filling your lungs to approximately two-thirds capacity.

Hold your breath for several seconds.

Exhale fully.

Repeat this cycle ten times.

This simple practice can shortcut the stress response in as little as one minute, depending on the intensity of your fight-or-flight condition. Even if you're in a situation in which breathing is socially unacceptable, such as at a business luncheon with tough-minded associates who have little regard for oxygen, you can still use this technique. Simply remain focused on your breathing while you continue to look at others and monitor the conversation at the table. They'll think you're listening to them attentively, but what you're doing is secretly stimulating parasympathetic dominance. It's really quite exciting.

By holding in the breath for several seconds the carotid bodies, tiny clumps of nerve tissue containing specialized chemical receptors and located along the carotid arteries, are fooled into thinking that blood pressure is rising. The carotid bodies will then signal a message for blood vessels to dilate, which causes an overall drop in blood pressure and hence a diminishment of the stress response.

By breathing in to only two-thirds of your lung capacity, you ensure that blood pressure won't go up from the sheer exertion of forcing the lungs to maximum expansion. By breathing out more fully than you breathe in, you help move stale air out from the lungs. Slow, deep breathing has also been shown to increase endorphin release in the body, producing a sense of relaxation and well-being.

With basic deep breathing it's preferable to breathe in and out through the nose. Air entering through the nasal passages is quickly warmed to body temperature because lungs work most efficiently with warm air. Step outside on a cold winter day, breathe in through your mouth, and you'll prove this to yourself quite easily as the cold air causes the lungs to tense. Nasal breathing also has a potent effect on the central nervous system because nerve receptors in the nose reach directly to the brain. If your sinuses are clogged and nasal breathing is difficult, breathing through the mouth will still work sufficiently.

A useful variation on this technique is to place a hand on your belly, or even one hand atop the other over your abdomen. This may help you focus more clearly on your gut and relax more deeply.

People often talk about burning calories but few realize that a calorie is simply a measure of heat released when something is burned. Food scientists determine the caloric value of a food by placing it in a special apparatus that essentially torches it to a crisp and measures the heat given off. It shouldn't surprise you, then, that just about everything has a measurable caloric value. A fortune cookie contains about thirty calories. This page you're reading has at least sixty calories. The chair you're sitting in has upward of one hundred thousand calories. And all of these calories need oxygen to burn.

If you want to maximize metabolism, breathing is one of the most effective tools because the greater your capacity to take in oxygen, the higher your metabolic "burning power" will be.

Breathe in more oxygen and you burn food more fully.

It's really that simple. The digestive system is hungry for oxygen. Certain parts of the stomach lining consume more oxygen than any other tissue in the body. The intestinal villi, our site of primary nutrient absorption, are charged with the job of extracting large quantities of oxygen from the blood during the breakdown of a meal. When the blood lacks oxygen for the villi to pick up, absorption decreases.

The more we eat, the more the body naturally wants us to breathe. After a meal, the parasympathetic nervous system initiates synchronous changes in breathing, blood circulation, and oxygen uptake. In other words, the brain automatically increases air intake to accommodate the need for more oxygen. Breathing more if you eat a lot is the same as exercising more if you eat a lot. If you interfere with the body's natural switch to deeper breathing because of anxiety or overstimulation, you limit your ability to burn calories. The simple rule here is this: If you eat more, breathe more.

To further examine the relationship between oxygen and weight loss, have you ever had the experience of going on a low-calorie diet and not losing any weight, or dieting and losing weight the first week but leveling off despite continuing your low-calorie fare? Many people are perplexed by this mysterious phenomenon, but the reason is quite simple. Your metabolism changed. The body learned to tolerate the meager portions of food you served it by lowering oxygen uptake—decreased oxygen means decreased metabolism. In many cases, weight-loss diets actually teach the body to need less oxygen. So by going on a low-calorie diet you may think you're doing what's right for shedding pounds, but you're actually working against yourself.

Another way to think of this phenomenon is to consider that the act of eating creates a "demand" on metabolism. Just as lifting weights puts a demand on your muscles to grow bigger and stronger, eating food puts a demand on your metabolism to grow more powerful and efficient. Food is literally like a weight that your body lifts. So it's not just the nutrients in the food that determine the nutritional and metabolic value of a meal; the value is also determined by the process your body goes through to break down the food.

Indeed, the simple act of eating, by itself, raises metabolism. If we looked at one of the most common measures of metabolism—body temperature—we'd see that each time we eat, body temperature automatically rises. That's the reality behind the old folk-medicine adage to "starve a fever"—if you already have a high body temperature, don't eat because that will raise it even more.

Can you see how starving yourself or eating meals that are too low in calories can be counterproductive to weight loss?

It should come as no surprise that if eating less food can lower the amount of oxygen we use, and hence lower the metabolism, then eating more food could increase metabolism. Indeed, many people I've worked with who honestly had weight to lose and were on a long-term, low-calorie diet without success lost their weight once they ate more food. Do you know someone who's had this unusual experience? Eating more food literally created a demand for metabolic force and hence for oxygen uptake. The resulting increase in calorie-burning capacity far "outweighed" the extra food on their plate.

Certainly, many of us gain weight simply because we eat too much food. But when we shift to the opposite extreme—eating too little food—we will likely slow down our calorie-burning capacity. On any given day approximately sixty million Americans are on a diet. If low-calorie diets—meaning 1,400 calories a day or less—were truly effective in the long-term, then we'd see a lot more success and a lot less dieters. The point is not to overeat and expect to lose weight. The point is that neither extreme—too much food or too little—will take you where you want to go.

Facts You Should Know About Vitamin O

One of the best-kept secrets in the nutrition business is this. There's only one true miracle nutrient, it has profound metabolic power, it's freely available and is seldom used to the fullest. The miracle nutrient is vitamin O—oxygen. And we need lots of it. With food, quality is what's important. With oxygen, quantity is what counts. Plenty of people restrict their eating intake but no one goes on an oxygen diet. Try it some time and see what happens. You can survive for four weeks without food, four days without water, but you can last only four minutes without oxygen. Talk about a highly essential nutrient! Whether you've known it or not, oxygen has been and always will be your number one nutritional priority.

The bottom line is that if you don't have breathing, you don't have a meal. The entire process of digestion is designed to break food down into microscopic morsels that can be sent to your cells and combusted with oxygen for energy release. Over 95 percent of all energy generated in the body comes from the simple combination of oxygen plus food. Without oxygen your food is literally useless. Start a fire in your fireplace and the two things that concern you most are good wood (fuel) and the right amount of air circulation. Without oxygen, the fire couldn't exist and the fuel wouldn't burn. The same is true for your body. Indeed, the body itself is literally a heat-producing biological machine. Just about every chemical reaction inside us has, as a by-product, heat. At the cellular level, then, food is the fuel, and oxygen literally serves to fan our metabolic flames. That's why the most commonly used measurement for metabolic rate is oxygen utilization. Metabolism is oxygen. And oxygen comes from breathing.

It's amazing how the breath is such a vital yet overlooked part of our diet. In junior high school biology most of us learned that oxygen combined with carbohydrates (food) yields energy release. Yet few of us learned the secret that when you breathe more, you burn more.

If you truly want to achieve your optimum weight and metabolism, you can't get there by denying yourself and going against biology. Losing weight means gaining life. Eat while relaxed and breathe with full generosity and you access nature's plan for greater health and inner satisfaction with food.

There's still more to the oxygen story. Increased oxygen not only helps us burn food but is also necessary for burning the body's own internal fuel source—fat. The "training effect" of any regular exercise yields two key benefits. First, exercise simply helps your body take in more oxygen. Second, your body learns how to use that oxygen better. And the body's strategy for a more efficient use of oxygen is to enlist body fat as a fuel. What's amazing is that you can get at least some of the benefits of aerobic exercise simply by training yourself to breathe more fully as you sit and eat. You'll also prosper in the fat-burning department if you remind yourself to breath more deeply throughout the day. Breathing is literally a fat-burning exercise!

Exercise: Breathe While You Eat

Breathing during meals is a great way to help you become a slow, relaxed eater. If you're eating while distracted by work tasks or involved in tense conversations, or if you're a habitually fast eater, your breathing will be more shallow. By reminding yourself to breathe more deeply during meals, you'll naturally slow down, become more present, and metabolize with greater power.

To increase your breath intake during eating, at least three times during any meal ask yourself "How is my breathing?" Then consciously deepen your breath with as little effort as possible. Focus on deep breathing to a level that's new for you yet still feels natural and comfortable.

Use gentle, fuller breathing as a natural pause during meals. Delight in oxygen as you would delight in the food itself. Deep breathe three times at each pause.

Consider the oxygen you inspire as fundamental to your meal as a salad or a pickle. With each deepened breath you'll deliver more oxygen into your bloodstream and to your cells, where it will instan-taneously generate greater calorie-burning power. After several weeks, you'll notice that breathing while you eat has become a new habit. You won't need to remind yourself as often because it will be a natural and automatic part of eating. By slowing down to breathe you will increase your metabolic speed.

Interestingly enough, another simple way you can increase your oxygen intake and hence your metabolism is by opening a window. The per-centage of oxygen in outdoor air is generally greater than indoor envi-ronments. A lack of oxygen in stale indoor air or windowless rooms—our typical workspace or office building—is a physiologic stressor to the body. When the quantity of oxygen in an indoor space is too low, heart rate and blood pressure slightly increase, and blood sugar drops; we feel drowsy, irritable, low energy, and in need of a boost. And what's the typical strategy we use when feeling this way? We reach for food or a cup of coffee to pick us up. Many of us hunger for oxygen but mistake it as a hunger for food.

As is often the case, it's the big-money people who truly make the best use of these medical realities. Next time you go to a Las Vegas casino and wonder how it is that people stay up all hours gambling with energy, enthusiasm, and abandon, you can thank oxygen. Rumor has it that the casinos pump extraordinary amounts of O_2 into their climate-controlled rooms to keep you alert. They use one vital commodity to relieve you of another. Can you imagine what our work life would be like if all busi-nesses and employers were as committed to maximum oxygenation as our friends in Las Vegas?

As you experiment with these breathing techniques, notice any changes in your after-meal energy level and your satisfaction quotient and any improvements in digestive complaints. You might also wish to pay attention to breathing during your day because deliberate, slow, deep breaths will further increase the oxygenation of the body, which translates into even greater metabolic strength.

It's also useful to notice any resistance you might have to relaxing and slowing down with meals. Oftentimes making this shift can be quite confrontational. It can bring up the parts of us that are seemingly beyond our control. The way we do food is the way we do life. Slowing down with meals, then, is symbolic of relaxing into our body, our career, our fears and desires, and anything life presents. It's about granting ourselves the right to share in the simplicity of joyous moments on Earth. It's about reclaiming our time, our dignity, and the sanctity of self-care. If you've been eating your meals in the fast lane, it's time to relax into the metabolism you were meant to have.

More Tips for Relaxed Eating and Deep Breathing

Light a candle at the table, play sweet music, decorate your eating environment with objects of beauty and mirth.

- If you eat out, choose a restaurant that has a relaxed and nourishing atmosphere. If you are eating take-out food, find a peaceful or celebratory place outdoors to enjoy your meal.

- Dine with eating companions who nourish and inspire you.

- Let your conversation be elevating and free of negativity or gossip.

- Notice your posture as you eat. A straight spine allows for fuller, deeper breaths.

- During your workday, take a breathing break. Go outside for some fresh air, even if only for a few minutes.

- Use eating as a time to let go of all worries and work. Use juicy and positive thoughts to assist you in assimilating nutrients and burning calories. If you insist, you can resume worrying and working once your relaxed and nourishing meal is complete.

Key Lessons

- When the stress response is activated digestion shuts down. When the relaxation response is activated digestion is in full force.

- Chronic low-level stress, via cortisol and insulin, decreases calorie-burning capacity. Weight gain can result.

- Worrying and anxiety generate a stress response. Weight gain can result.

- The stress state creates the metabolic conditions for bone loss. A relaxed state supports bone health.

- Conscious breathing dissipates the stress response and promotes full digestive power.

- Oxygen is the most fundamental and necessary metabolic nutrient for the body. The more we breathe, the more we digest, assimilate, and calorie burn.

- Time is an essential nutrient.

- Before you focus on *what* to eat, teach yourself *how* to eat.

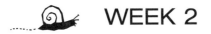 **WEEK 2**

The Metabolic Power of Quality

The discovery of a new dish does more for the happiness
of mankind than the discovery of a new star.

JEAN BRILLAT-SAVARIN

The biggest and most urgent nutritional question of our time—"What should I eat?"—happens to have the greatest assortment of confusing and contradictory answers. Fortunately I have a very practical suggestion on how you can become your own dietary expert and be assured of consistently making excellent nutritional choices, if not the best choices. If you allowed me the honor of being your personal nutritionist for just one dietary change, if you asked me "What's the one simple nutritional strategy that could give me the biggest bang for my metabolic buck, improve my health and weight more than any other change, and make a positive impact on the lives of others and the Earth itself?" here's the guideline I'd urge you to follow.

Elevate the quality of your food.

Quality is everything. In every major nutritional study that's ever been done comparing the diets of industrialized nations—mostly consisting of refined, mass-produced, poor-quality food—with the diets of

43

traditional cultures—fresh, whole, locally cultivated and vibrant—those on traditional diets fare dramatically better in every major health category.[1] Elevate the quality of your food and you elevate metabolism.

Quality means any or all of the following: real; fresh; organic; gourmet; lovingly crafted; homemade; locally produced; heirloom varieties; nutrient dense; low in human-made toxins; grown and marketed with honesty and integrity; tasteful; filled with true flavor, not virtual ones that mask the absence of nutrients and vitality. *Quality* means that care and consciousness permeate a food, and that the food itself has a good story to tell.

As it is with cars and other durable goods, with food you get what you pay for. Would you expect a car manufactured with the cheapest parts, hastily assembled and designed without any care for the needs of the driver to give you the ride of your life? Science doesn't have a way to measure the value and the effects of the quality of food on the human body because we still have our training wheels on in the nutrition business and can only maneuver ourselves around nutrient values. When we nutrition experts lay down the law about how the value of a food is gloriously revealed in its nutrient profile, it all sounds so scientific. And it is. Except that this measure of a meal's true worth is woefully limited and scientifically incomplete.

When the artistry of food is finally elevated to its rightful place, then the science will speak with more wisdom and clarity. What I'm talking about is not so much a different way of seeing food and nutrition as it is a whole new approach to the world and our place in it.

When science studies food, nutrition, or a supplement, it rarely looks at quality. That's a hidden reason behind why the results of food studies often conflict and why you're invariably fed contradictory messages about eating. Recall the famous "French paradox" discussed in the previous chapter—and how Europeans can eat a significantly greater amount of fat without the same rise in cholesterol level and heart disease that we Americans experience. Not only is this a function of the benefits Europeans receive from the metabolic power of relaxing, breathing, and taking their time with their meals, it's also about quality.

Much of the European cuisine is of a level that is worth aspiring to. This higher quality means a healthier metabolism. The only "paradox" here is why researchers couldn't see the big picture.

There's still another very important rationale for choosing high-quality foods that most of the experts tend to overlook, and one that certainly deserves your attention if you are concerned about weight: The poorer the quality of our food, the more quantity we'll consume.

The problem with overeating in our nation is not that we have a collective willpower disorder. Yes, many of us eat too much. But we do so, to a great degree, because our food is nutrient deficient. It lacks the vitamins, minerals, enzymes, and all the undiscovered x-factors and energies we require. The brain senses these deficiencies and wisely responds to this absence of vital chemistry by commanding us to undertake the most sensible survival strategy: eat more food. If a movie or a party you attended lacked substance, you'd walk away feeling unfulfilled and wanting more. It's the same with food.

By choosing organic foods, your diet becomes more nutrient dense. That's because pound for pound, organic foods have more vitamins and minerals than their inorganic and mass-produced counterparts. They also have less xenotoxins—humanmade substances such as pesticides and herbicides that function as antinutrients and disease agents. Organic simply means "real."

Of course, it's easy to become apathetic when hearing endless messages about the carcinogens in our food, the evils of carbohydrates, or the mercury in fish. I often hear people lament "Everything's bad for you." But now you have a powerful tool to help bust through such nutritional confusion:

**No matter what food you eat, choose
the highest quality version of that food.**

This gives you the best Las Vegas odds that the food will be healthy, whether you're eating bacon, bananas, bread, or birthday cake. Yes, quality foods are definitely more expensive. But this is the *real* health insurance. It's your life we're talking about, yours and those of the loved ones you feed.

Food Is . . .

Before we look at specific suggestions on how to include quality foods in our diet, let's better understand the true metabolic power of quality by examining more closely what food really is.

Most people would say that food is a collection of vitamins, minerals, macronutrients, and other chemicals. To determine the value of a meal, we'd measure the amount of nutrients it contains—read any product label and you'll see this philosophy in action. But it's time to catch up with the new millennium. This view of food is no longer adequate in describing nutritional reality. Food is much more than a bunch of chemicals. Food is energy and information.

This definition applies to any substance we consume, be it water, an herb, a supplement, a drug, caviar, or cotton candy. Whatever metabolic effect the body receives from any of these happens because that substance communicated a specific message to our cells. The caffeine in coffee literally tells the heart to beat faster and our blood pressure to spike and instructs the nervous system to accelerate its functions. The fiber in your oatmeal actually chats with your intestines, telling them to contract, and has a side conversation with your liver, pancreas, and bloodstream, asking your LDL cholesterol to drop and your blood sugar to stabilize. The bioflavonoids in your berries instruct the body to keep tiny blood vessels strong and supple, to reduce cellular inflammation, and to slow down the aging process of specific tissues such as the macula of the eyes. Food talks to your body and your body talks back.

This is not a fanciful notion about metabolism; it is a scientific reality. With his simple formula $E=MC^2$, Einstein proved that matter and energy are one and the same and could shapeshift to and fro. And both are loaded with information. Indeed, every speck of creation—from a humble particle of dust to a galactic sun—holds vast quantities of information, also called memory. Simply because we can't always perceive with our five senses this hidden library within all matter doesn't mean it's not there.

Consider, for example, the tomato. If the soil it grows in is depleted, then the tomato has measurably low mineral content, less natural sugar, and more acids, which means it will be tough, tasteless, and nutritionally inferior. If it is sprayed with pesticides and herbicides, it will carry instructional messages to your body that are carcinogenic, mutagenic, and neurotoxic. If it is grown on an impersonal factory farm, the tomato will be lifeless and have no charm. If it is picked by an underpaid migrant worker who's given no benefits and few worker's rights, then the tomato is hypocritical and lacks integrity. If it is chopped by machine along with thousands of other tomatoes, delivered to a fast-food joint, and slapped together with a bun and meat from a cow who suffered even worse traumas, then our tomato is now suicidal, or even murderous, because it has lost its soul and has no reason to live. I think you get the picture.

Ancient healing systems such as Ayurveda and Chinese medicine have long recognized the energetic nature of food. Rather than describe the chemical elements of a meal, these approaches look at the "archetypal" elements. They see earth, water, wood, fire, and metal; kapha, pitta, and vata; yin and yang. None of these elements are seen under a microscope but they are plainly observed in action, much the way our character is revealed for all to see yet is nowhere to be found. Yin and yang are as real to the Chinese as proteins and fats are to us.

The true worth of a food, then, will never be discerned from a label. Its real value is in all the energy and information it contains. Yes, that includes vitamin, mineral, protein, fiber, and fat content. But it also means how the food is grown, handled, transported, manufactured, advertised, cooked, served, and eaten. All this information lives inside a food as surely as you live inside your body.

So if we want to truly quell the rise of heart disease with the help of diet, then it's time to put more heart into how we create food, eat it, and share it with the hungry. If we want to slow the unchecked growth of cancerous cells in the human family and limit the amount of carcinogens in our food, then it's time to slow down the world, take stock of *our* unchecked growth, and rethink the manic way that we manufacture our nourishment.

Many people want food to provide them with health, happiness, and all the blessings of beauty. Well, the only way food can possibly deliver such a huge bounty is if we create it in that image. When the energies of love and beauty are cultivated into a foodstuff, such will be our harvest.

Limiting the Antinutrients in Your Diet

When it comes to empowered eating, it's as important to ease off of the antinutritious foods as it is to include the healthy ones. Antinutrients literally break down the body's metabolic machinery at the cellular level. The most potent antinutrients to limit are:

- Poor-quality fats
- Poor-quality sugar
- Poor-quality white flour
- Poor-quality dairy
- Poor-quality meats

Poor-quality fat means any food that contains hydrogenated oil, partially hydrogenated oil, hydrogenated palm kernel oil, margarine and any margarine-like spreads with hydrogenated oil, cottonseed oil, Olestra (a synthetic fat), and most commercial supermarket-bought cooking oils. Poor-quality fat also includes most fried foods—french fries, chicken, chips, and so forth.

Read the labels on everything you buy. Hydrogenated oils are found in many mass-produced food products, including potato chips, corn chips, crackers, cookies, prepared foods, frozen foods, baked goods, snacks, and others. Most of the oils you find in a supermarket are highly processed—heated at high temperatures and stripped of their sensitive essential fats and other nutrients.

As best as you can, replace poor-quality fat-containing products with quality oils and quality-fat foods.

These would include olive oil, sesame oil, and coconut oil—all of these oils are great for cooking. Other oils to use for dressings and dips include sunflower, flaxseed, hazelnut, pistachio, hempseed, and macadamia nut oils. Always use expertly processed unrefined organic oils—these can generally be found at a health food store. (As a side note, I'm not a big fan of canola oil. It's not very heat stable and most brands are overprocessed. The same goes for soy oil.)

Use real butter rather than margarine—the best choices are hormone free and farm fresh or organic. Butter made from raw and unpasteurized milk is best. Ghee can be used as a substitute for butter. Ghee is clarified butter, also called separated butter; it is a traditional, time-tested food from India that is highly heat stable and so can be used for browning or light frying.

Other preferred sources of health-giving fats include:

Avocado—organic and fresh is best

Olives—emphasize variety

Fresh fish—especially those that are ocean or stream caught and not farm raised; focus on variety

Nuts and seeds—organic is always best

Nut butter—peanut butter, almond butter, sesame butter

Free-range eggs—eggs that come from a real chicken running around a real farm eating real food

Organic dairy products—especially those that are produced from raw and unpasteurized milk from grass-fed animals, including yogurt, cheese, and milk

By the way, healthy fat in your food does not translate to fat on your body. If you deprive yourself of essential fat to lose weight, you'll get the opposite result. And even if you lose weight, you'll likely suffer from some of the symptoms of clinical fat deficiency—irritability, fatigue, dull and brittle hair, dry skin, redness around the eyes, digestive complaints, constipation, inability to lose weight, and mood disorders. So on behalf of all the nutritionists, dieticians, and doctors who have been feeding you the wrong information since the late 1960s, I'd like to apologize. It's not your fault that we sent you down the wrong road. Remember, this is the same group of well-intentioned experts that invented hospital food. We mean well but we don't always hit the mark.

Fat is essential to life to such a degree that if we could suck all the fat out of your body—the ultimate liposuction service—you'd die in an instant. Fat serves as an energy source for the heart and brain. It's a building block for many of the hormones and chemicals that keep us alive. It's a nutritional source for the central nervous system, and it lines and protects every organ. For these reasons and more, and because the body cannot produce on its own all the specific fats we require, we have labeled such important components of our diet "essential fats," also known as "essential fatty acids" or "EFAs." You might also have heard them called "omega-3" and "omega-6" fatty acids as well.

Fat serves a most profound structural function—it's a building block for the wall of every cell in your body. The walls of your cells are in no way similar to the walls in your house. An architectural wall is stiff, solid, unintelligent, impermeable to the elements, and can be made of anything that keeps the outside from coming in and the inside from leaking out.

Our cell walls are the exact opposite. They are pliable, permeable, highly complex, and extremely intelligent—to the point where they must precisely control the traffic of thousands of kinds of biomolecules across their surface each millisecond. When it comes to the body, the cell wall is where the rubber meets the road, so to speak, and healthy fat is an indispensable part of the process.

Perhaps the ultimate kudos for fat is that it comprises approximately 40 to 60 percent of your brain. How's that for an unsexy statistic? So the next time you think, you have fat to thank.

In small quantities, of course, poor-quality fats are harmless to most people. But when poor-quality fats become part of our staple fare, day in and day out, our health will eventually suffer. These fats, which are chemically different from the quality kind, literally become the building blocks of our cell wall. The result is that the cell wall becomes more rigid, susceptible to oxidation (rusting or aging), and less intelligent—it loses its ability to make smart choices about what goes in and what comes out. This is a special concern when it comes to the brain, which is largely composed of essential omega-3 fat. When poor-quality fat is incorporated into its structure, brain tissue is more easily oxidized and becomes biologically stiff (and thus stupid). This will make you less interesting at parties, as well as increasing the probability of Alzheimer's, dementia, and other brain diseases. Including more healthy fat and cutting down on the dysfunctional ones is, therefore, a "no brainer."

Poor-quality sugar refers to any food that contains high-fructose corn syrup, fructose corn syrup, corn syrup, white sugar, glucose, Florida Crystals, or any artificial sweetener. Read product labels to reveal these ingredients. The various forms of corn syrup are commonly found in soft drinks, juice drinks, sweet candies, and packaged snack foods and cookies, and even in the so-called "healthy" protein bars. As best you can, eliminate products with these ingredients from your home. Let them be an occasional exception on your menu rather than the rule.

Replace commercial sodas and soft drinks with organic juices, herbal ice teas, or water. With variety as the key, use organic jams; fresh fruit; organic or fresh cookies, pastries, and muffins; organic candies; organic ice creams and sorbets.

Replace all "reward foods" with higher quality health-food-store versions that use quality sweeteners such as the following.

Raw honey: The jar must say "raw" or "unheated" on the label. Raw honey is high in enzymes and phytochemicals related to plants and their pollens. It is traditionally used as both food and medicine. Raw honey is not suitable for infants.

Maple syrup: High in minerals and phytochemicals. Organic varieties of maple syrup are free of the formaldehyde used in most mass-produced products.

Barley malt: Less sweet than other sweeteners; good for baking.

Stevia: A noncaloric all-natural herbal sweetener with medicinal properties. A small amount can sweeten your beverage or tea.

The scientific "party line" states that all sugars—be they white sugar, corn syrup, honey, maple syrup, and so on—are essentially the same from a chemical standpoint. Unfortunately, there is no current scientific model that is subtle and accurate enough to reveal the true distinctions between these vastly different packages of energy and information. Consequently, our collective diet is top-heavy with an excess of poor-quality sweeteners, and we suffer the consequences—obesity, heart disease, and diabetes.

By the way, you might think that diet sodas and artificial sweeteners would help us lose weight because they contain no calories and no sugar to spike our insulin. But this isn't really the case. After forty years of exposure to fake chemical sweeteners, not a single study has ever shown an even mildly convincing association between sugar substitutes and weight loss.

Instead, researchers are now discovering that artificial sweeteners—fake pleasure—may actually cause us to gain weight. As fate would have it, the artificial sweetener molecule is so crafty that it convinces the brain that it's real sugar, so the body releases insulin to help metabolize the artificial sugar. Since there is no real sugar present, the excess insulin, with nothing to do, performs its other evolutionary task, which is to signal the body to store fat. As well, there is firmly mounting evidence that aspartame is a significant neurotoxin. So my professional advice to you is this: If you have any synthetically sweetened foods in your home, step on them to ensure you kill them, then toss them out.

Poor-quality white flour means products such as mass-produced pastas, breads, cookies, muffins, and bagels; crackers; cold breakfast cereals;

sugar-sweetened oatmeal products; commercial granola bars; pretzels, pastries, and donuts.

It's only in the past century that our diet has included such a large amount of refined and highly processed carbohydrates—white flour products, breads, cookies, donuts, chips, pretzels, cereals, crackers, pasta, sweets, and so on. Our ancestors ate carbohydrate foods in their unprocessed state. When we consume these foods, which have been stripped of most of their vitamin and mineral contents, our insulin level shoots up too high, which signals the body to store weight and store fat. Excess insulin also causes the body to crave even more sugar and more carbohydrate foods. Diabetes, heart disease, and a host of degenerative diseases can follow.

An assortment of diet books, like those espousing the Atkins diet, the Zone diet, Sugar Busters, Paleolithic diets, high-protein diets, and others, all have one common and very useful nugget of wisdom at their core—too many refined carbohydrates in our diet is problematic. So rather than concern yourself with the precise amount of carbohydrates your body scientifically needs (hint: no such assessment exists anyway), begin your exploration of the metabolic power of quality by including the carbohydrates that have a quality story to tell and limiting or eliminating as best you can those that don't. This alone will begin to curb carbohydrate cravings and significantly assist you in discovering your body's natural intelligence in determining portions, percentages, and amounts.

Look through your home and begin to replace poor-quality white-flour products with quality carbohydrate foods.

These would include organic varieties of brown rice, beans, quinoa, barley, corn, amaranth, oats, oatmeal, lentils, chickpeas, millet (grains and beans are best when presoaked before cooking); organic and/or fresh-made pastas; sourdough or sprouted breads or fresh whole-grain breads; rye crackers; crackers free of hydrogenated oils; organic chips (corn, potato, and rice chips without oil or made with olive oil); organic vegetables, including squash, sweet potato, yam, root vegetables, potato;

organic fruit, with variety as the key.

If you're looking to cut down on carbohydrates, your focus should be on the refined, mass-produced kind. And it's a great idea to consider limiting the amount of gluten in your diet—which is primarily found in any product containing wheat. Vegetables are fine. High-starch vegetables are also fine, just go easy on them. Fruits are also great—just make sure you focus on variety and don't limit your fruit to pineapples, grapes, bananas, and dried fruit, as these can be quite high in natural sugar. Whole grains such as brown rice are preferable to their white cousins, but as a nutritionist I will tell you that it's also no big deal to have white rice or white bread from time to time. As long as these are not major staple foods in your diet, I've never heard of anyone dying from their occasional consumption.

Poor-quality dairy means mass-produced, nonorganic, hormone-containing cheese, milk, yogurt, cream cheese, cottage cheese, flavored milks, and snack foods with cheese by-products.

The days of the exalted position of milk and cheese in our diet is numbered. Evidence is mounting that milk's preeminence as a source of absorbable calcium is way overstated and perhaps even untrue. Look to leafy greens and nuts and seeds as excellent sources of bioavailable calcium. In addition to lactose intolerance (an inability to metabolize milk sugar), many people are sensitive or highly allergic to the protein component of milk without realizing it. When the protein in milk undergoes high-temperature heating, as it does in pasteurization, the complex milk protein molecule—casein—is radically altered, which can render it cytotoxic and neurotoxic. If you experience any combination of chronic sinus complaints, nasal or lung congestion, postnasal drip, digestive sensitivity, headaches, multiple allergies, and dry skin, you are a great candidate to experiment with a diet free of all milk and dairy-containing products during week 2. Even if you don't have these symptoms, I would highly recommend that you try dairy-free eating during this time and see what that change does for you.

Nutrition experts continually disagree about the merits of milk and dairy foods. That's because most of the commercially available products in this category are of extremely poor quality.

In general, I suggest you keep dairy foods to a minimum. When you do use dairy products, replace mass-produced, poor-quality varieties with the following.

Milk: Raw, organic, and unpasteurized is best. Locally produced with no hormones is a plus.

Cheese: Organic, or any high-quality locally produced or imported varieties made from raw and unpasteurized milk.

Yogurt: Full fat, organic, or locally produced when possible.

Cottage cheese: Full fat, organic, and fresh is best.

Butter: Local varieties, organic, raw milk, and European imports are generally the highest quality.

You can also use rice milk, almond milk, soy yogurt, rice yogurt, and soy- and rice-based ice creams as dairy-free substitutes.

Poor-quality meat refers to all fast-food meats; processed meats such as packaged cold cuts and commercially produced hot dogs; meats in frozen prepared foods; any fresh or frozen meat that isn't free range, hormone free, and fed real food; any meat produced from animals that are not raised and slaughtered with care and humanity.

As best as you can, replace these poor-quality meats with any chicken, turkey, beef, pork, lamb, or other meat or poultry that is labeled free range, organic, grass fed, or hormone free.

Many such products can be found fresh at your supermarket or deli. You can also find organically produced hot dogs, hamburgers, chicken soups, sausages, and other popular frozen and prepared meat items at a well-stocked health food store. Free-range eggs (sometimes called omega eggs) are the preferred quality choice. You can also replace some or all of the meat in your diet with fresh or smoked fish or vegetarian sources of protein such as tofu, tempeh, and nut butters.

It's high time that we get real about our meat eating. Humankind owes its survival, in great part, to the animals we've eaten. To argue that meat eating is wrong negates the sustenance that has enabled us to be here so we could have something to argue about in the first place. And yet our overreliance on animal foods is clearly imbalanced and our relation to the animal kingdom is killing us. Our drive to mass produce meat is dramatically polluting our environment and stealing away valuable land and water from developing nations. It's also making our cows "mad." The inescapable truth is that eating a creature raised and sacrificed without honor and care invokes disease upon the human family.

It might interest you to know that the most expensive and highly prized meat on Earth comes to us courtesy of the Kobe cows. These are quality bovines and their desirability has everything to do with lifestyle. In fact, if you're ever needing to feel jealous toward a group of cows, these are the ones you should focus on. The Kobe cows live in Hawaii. They enjoy perfect weather and sunshine, they eat the healthiest, tastiest grass grown on nutrient-rich volcanic soil, they breathe fresh island air and have a beautiful ocean view, and they are blessed with plenty of time for socializing and quiet reflection. They're living the dream. Is it any wonder they taste so good? You would too.

The point is that these cows feed back to the eater exactly what was given to them: life, harmony, nourishment, nutrition. Of course, when we contrast this with the dismal existence of factory-farmed animals it becomes apparent why the experts see such different results and draw so many contradictory conclusions about the relative health merits of meat.

The research varies because the quality of the meat varies. Consequently, some experts give their "thumbs up" to meat while others point the other way.[2] To me, the most compelling research shows that countries with a high per capita consumption of commercial meat products coupled with excessive refined carbohydrates, hydrogenated fats, and poor-quality vegetable oils show the highest "meat-associated" cancer rates, whereas in traditional societies with no sugar, white-flour products, or poor-quality oils but with high-quality meats, no association between cancer and meat eating exists.[3] Can you see the implications?

Week 2: Your Primary Task

Week 2 is your opportunity to do the best you can in cleaning out the low-end, mass-produced, unenlightened food products from your home and replacing them with high-quality counterparts. It's a time to focus on food that is fresh or home cooked, organic, locally grown, and is the best you can find given whatever factors may limit you—time, convenience, money, or availability. During this time, let go of your need to know exactly which foods to eat and how much.

Your primary task in week 2, then, is this: Whenever and whatever you eat, hit the target at least 80 percent of the time with quality food choices. This assures that you'll be receiving the nutrients you require to thrive while eliminating the toxic substances that pollute the food web and suppress metabolic potential. Think of week 2 as a new beginning in how you value the nourishment of your body. Celebrate this fresh start by knowing that you're raising the bar in how you honor the miracle of sustenance that connects us all. Say goodbye to the foods that fail to reflect the quality, taste, and vitality you deserve and welcome the ones that do. This doesn't mean you can never eat a marshmallow or an English muffin again. It simply means that the overall direction of your diet is quality, that you're choosing to bring a higher level of food into the sanctity of your home, and that anything other than quality is the exception and not the rule.

Let's be real. Most of us are going to stray from what we know is "healthy." At some point, we *will* eat the cake, the cookies, the pasta, and the junk. We *will* drink the alcohol. So be it. Let's just make that part of our nutrition program rather than pretend it isn't. That's the middle way, the honest way, and for many people, the practical way. And in this day and age, it may well be the healthiest way. Really. So don't waste your energy trying to be a saint and then demonize yourself when sainthood inevitably fails. If at least 80 percent of the food that passes your lips is high quality, you'll be doing fine. Anything more is a welcome bonus.

Exercise: Quality Shopping

During week 2, find out the location of the most well stocked natural foods supermarkets or food cooperatives in your area. Some of the big chains include Wild Oats, Whole Foods, Wild By Nature, and Trader Joes. Many of these stores have a section of freshly prepared natural foods for those of us with little time to cook.

Set aside several hours to walk through the store. Explore, read labels, ask questions, and see what foods catch your attention. Do the best you can in switching over to organic fare.

If you have young children, bring them along to shop and include them in the process. Tell them your nutritionist said that if they want to grow big and strong or have nice skin and shiny hair, eating good food is the way to go. Give them choices from the snack sections or prepared foods and let them feel empowered in participating in their new lifestyle.

Also, identify the best places to purchase healthy meats, fresh fish, fresh whole-grain or sourdough breads, and locally grown organic produce. Create a shopping schedule that assures healthy, high-quality food is always at home this week. In other words, don't let shopping be a haphazard affair. Prioritize it and make it a special ritual.

Remember, you are looking to shift to the most quality choices of the foods you are going to eat anyway. If you must have potato chips, buy an organic variety that is baked and made with olive oil. If you're going to drink coffee, go organic and forget the artificial sweeteners. If you absolutely want bagels, buy the freshest. If you drink juice, squeeze your own oranges, buy a juicer, or purchase organic brands, especially for your kids. If you're going to use canned or frozen foods, use organic brands. It's all about making the best possible choices given the choices you're going to make anyway. Apply this thinking to anything you eat and you'll be way ahead on the nutritional curve for health.

But Please, Just Tell Me What to Eat

As you're noticing, this is a diet program that doesn't tell you exactly which foods to eat and in what amounts. This is the greatest favor I can do for you as a nutritionist. Empowering you to be in deeper relationship with food and with the genius in your body is the surest road to your most powerful metabolism.

If you absolutely insist that you must know the precise and eternally correct answer to the question "What should I eat?" I have an important piece of advice: Let it go. Save your sanity. The quest for the perfect diet that will make us happy, healthy, and glamorous forever has created some heavy burdens we no longer need carry. Many people bounce from diet to diet and from one expert to the next often feeling victimized by the conflicting messages spoken by our food gurus and clueless about what to do. It's time to understand the territory.

The field of nutrition is frontier land. It's the Wild West. That's just the way it is. Many of the nutritional assertions we experts hold dear have a brief shelf life and will soon be replaced by something more crispy and fresh. That's because the science of eating is always changing, just like you and me. We are still discovering who we are and what sustains us. Perhaps this will always be so.

So rather than feeling discouraged by the endless amount of conflicting and difficult-to-follow nutrition information that the experts put forth, relax into the middle way. Let quality be your most trustworthy guide. Yes, there are specific foods and amounts that are the best and most beneficial for you to eat. But such information is not found in any book or revealed by any expert. It's found inside you. It's a practice of attunement that comes with time. That's what this program is about.

You'll learn more about how to discover the foods and their quantities that are right for you in the next chapter. For now, quality nutrition is your first and most fundamental step. Elevating food quality is the most practical and foolproof nutritional improvement you can make. And it has repercussions that are beautiful and far-reaching. For health is not an individual issue localized to your metabolism alone. It extends outward from the body as far as we can see and well beyond. Disregarding the Earth, its soil, and the food web and not thoughtfully sharing with all our fellow eaters around the planet has pathological consequences, not the least of which is recorded in our food as energy and information and fed directly back to us.

What goes around comes around. That's not a fanciful notion but a literal nutritional fact. Whatever it is you want a food to gift you with is yours to have, provided those same gifts have been bestowed upon the food. This may be, perhaps, the greatest nutritional secret of our time.

Key Lessons

- Eating quality food is perhaps the most powerful and foolproof nutritional strategy we can choose.

- Higher-quality food means greater nutritional value. When we continually eat low-quality food, the brain will register a nutrient deficit and signal us to eat more.

- Many people who think they have a willpower problem are experiencing a lack of nutrient-dense food.

- No matter what food you eat, choose the highest quality version of that food.

- First and foremost, food is energy and information.

- Every experience in the history of a food is encoded within it as energy and information. This is a significant determinant in its nutritional value.

More Tips for Quality Eating and Living

At the beginning of the week, make a list in your journal of everything that would stand in the way of including quality food in your life: "Not enough time," "It's too expensive," "My partner [or my kids] won't go for it," "No convenient healthy places to shop," "The food won't taste as good."

Then methodically and creatively uncover ways to help circumvent these concerns. Identify all the quality restaurants and takeout establishments near where you live and work. If you eat Japanese food, who has the freshest and the best? Mexican? Chinese? Who has the best salad bar? Homemade soups? If you're going to eat pizza, eat the best slice in town. If you order food in when you're at work, make the decision to make the best choices in regard to quality and freshness.

Quality also counts when it comes to water. Invest in a water filter for your kitchen and use for both drinking and cooking.

Almost anything placed on our skin will make its way into the body. That's why I recommend using skincare products that you can almost eat. Consider changing over the following products to natural and more environment-friendly varieties: soap, shampoo, conditioner, moisturizer, cosmetics, deodorant, shaving gel, toothpaste, and mouthwash. A health food store or food coop is the best resource for natural brands.

Quality household products also support health and ease the toxic load that humans have been continuously subjected to for the past century. As best as you can, replace dishwashing soap, all cleaners, laundry detergents, bleach, drain cleaners, and so forth with more earth-friendly varieties. Again, a well-stocked health-food store or food cooperative is an excellent place to find such products.

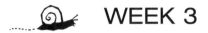 **WEEK 3**

The Metabolic Power of Awareness

Awareness cures.

Fritz Perls

One of the most unusual scientific revelations of the last century is the mathematical proof that the act of observing any phenomenon in the universe—be it the flight of a bird or the rotation of a planet—has a direct influence upon that phenomenon. According to the laws of physics, we have no choice but to alter the bird's course or the planet's speed simply by focusing our awareness on it. So if we have the power to tweak the orbit of a heavenly body, it should come as no surprise that vitamin A—awareness—also has a profound impact on the human body.

Have you ever looked in the mirror, liked what you saw, and suddenly felt your mood elevate and your energy perk up? That's awareness sparking the chemistry of metabolism. Have you ever been somewhere in nature, taking in the beauty of your surroundings, and felt an immediate and deep sense of relaxation? That's also awareness acting upon the physiology of the body. Or have you ever noticed when being watched that you seem to perform and express yourself with greater energy and focus? That's the awareness of others impacting your biochemistry.

Awareness is presence. It's our ability to be awake to what is. It's our capacity to experience what life is doing in this moment. And when we bring awareness to our eating experience, it's a wondrous metabolic force.

Digestion Begins in the Mind

The power of awareness to catalyze nutrient assimilation, digestion, and calorie-burning ability is best exemplified in something scientists call cephalic phase digestive response—CPDR. Cephalic means "of the head." CPDR is simply a fancy term for the pleasures of taste, aroma, satisfaction, and the visual stimulation of a meal. In other words, it's the "head phase" of digestion. What's amazing is that researchers have estimated that as much as 30 to 40 percent of the total digestive response to any meal is due to CPDR—our full awareness of what we're eating.[1]

Can you recall a time when you saw your favorite food and your mouth started watering or your stomach began churning? That's the cephalic phase digestive response. Digestion quite literally begins in the head as chemical and mechanical receptors on the tongue and the oral and nasal cavities are stimulated by smelling food, tasting it, chewing it, and noticing it. A hearty awareness of our meal initiates the secretion of saliva, gastric acid and enzymes, gut-associated neuropeptides, and production of the full range of pancreatic enzymes, including trypsin, chymotrypsin, pancreatic amylase, and lipase. In addition, it causes blood to rush to the digestive organs, the stomach and intestines to rhythmically contract, and electrolyte concentrations throughout the digestive tract to shift in preparation for incoming food.

Awareness is metabolism.

So let's do the math. If scientists say that 30 to 40 percent of our total digestive response to any meal is due to CPDR, and if we choose not to be aware of our meal—that is, if we "fall asleep at the plate" and fail to register any sense of taste, smell, satisfaction, or visual interest—then we are metabolizing our meal at only 60 to 70 percent efficiency.

Lack of attention translates into decreased blood flow to the digestive organs, which, as we've seen, means less oxygenation and hence a weakened metabolic force. With less enzymatic output in the gut we become susceptible to digestive upset, bowel disorders, lowered immunity, and fatigue.

Are you beginning to see why "sleepwalking" through a meal is an ill-informed nutritional choice?

When You Eat, Eat

Here are encapsulations of some of my favorite research studies that illustrate the nutritional power of awareness.

The first involves something called "dichotomous listening."[2] Test subjects are asked to concentrate as two people talk simultaneously—one person speaks into your left ear about intergalactic space travel while the other chats in your right ear about the joys of financial planning. If you've had the experience of listening on the telephone while someone nearby in the kitchen starts talking as if you had the superhuman ability to be in two conversations at once, then you know what this feels like.

During a relaxed state, test subjects consumed a mineral drink. Absorption was measured in the small intestines for two minerals—sodium and chloride. They assimilated at 100 percent. When the same individuals were exposed to dichotomous listening and then given their nutrient drink, they showed a complete shutdown in sodium and chloride assimilation that lasted for up to one hour afterward. In other words, there was 0 percent absorbtion. The simple act of attending to two stimuli at once dramatically altered their metabolism.

In an Italian study on digestion and mental stimulation,[3] university students were shown a short film. Using electrogastrographic (EGG) methods, researchers could determine each student's digestive activity before viewing the film and during. A snack eaten before the film stimulated normal digestive contractions. But with a snack eaten during the movie, EGG rates dropped. This means gut motility decreased, which translates to lower enzymatic output and inefficient digestion. With lowered gut motility, food takes a longer time to traverse through the body, which can lead to autotoxicity—the production of irritable and poisonous substances being released into the bloodstream.

So if viewing a film or listening to several people at once can depreciate your metabolic bank account, what do you think happens when you eat and watch TV? Or when you eat while driving? Or when you eat while working at your desk? Metabolizing a meal is like absorbing a conversation. If you were talking with a friend and she didn't pay any attention, you'd walk away feeling incomplete and wishing for more. The essence of your exchange would have been minimally assimilated at best. The same goes with food.

More Awareness, Less Appetite

Have you ever had the experience of eating a good-sized meal, not paying much attention to it, and after finishing noticed that your belly felt full but your mouth was still hungry? Have you ever wondered why the body would behave in such a strange way by giving you this mixed message?

Well, the cephalic phase digestive response is not only a response; it's a full-blown nutritional requirement. The brain *must* experience taste, pleasure, aroma, and satisfaction so it can accurately assess a meal and catalyze our most efficient digestive force. When we eat too fast or fail to notice our food, the brain interprets this missed experience as hunger. It's not smart enough to say to us "Hey, you inhaled your breakfast, ate like a maniac during lunch, and snacked like a hungry beast. You don't need any more food." The brain simply says "I don't remember eating anything. I didn't get any satisfaction. Nothing happened. I'm hungry."

And so we reach for more food.

That's why about nine out of ten people I speak to who say they have an overeating problem don't. Their problem is that they don't eat when they eat. They have little awareness of their meals and fail to satisfy their CPDR requirement, which results in a continued longing for food. What's ironic is that those who fall into this category think they have a willpower problem. But they don't—actually, lack of willpower is just a minor player in their overeating. Drug companies spend millions researching and developing new appetite-suppressing compounds while unsuspecting eaters exert great effort to control their desire for food, and it's all a monumental misuse of energy. So if you've been beating yourself up because you think you've failed in the willpower department, it's time to call off the dogs.

Simply put, the less awareness you bring to the table, the more you'll need to eat and the greater your weight gain will be.

It's clear, then, that our appetite is genetically designed to be fulfilled rather than suppressed. So why not give up a war that can never be won—attacking your need to eat—and achieve a metabolic victory by doing the opposite of what you've been taught? Give your body and soul exactly what they want—an experience of eating that's rich in the fruits of awareness—and you'll never need to fight yourself again.

Your Thoughts May Be Fattening

Have you ever heard someone say "Just thinking about food makes me gain weight"? Amazingly enough, this may well be true. Scientists have described an interesting component of CPDR, something they call the cephalic phase insulin response. As we've seen, insulin is a hormone we produce to help metabolize carbohydrates or sugars in our meal. When you eat foods such as pasta, bread, muffins, cookies, cake, cereal, crackers, juice, or candy, you produce insulin quite readily. Insulin also has another interesting function. In excess amounts it signals the body to store fat and to inhibit muscle growth.

The cephalic phase insulin response is a measurable phenomenon where the body produces insulin when you simply look at a piece of cake or fantasize about a bowl of pasta. The digestion of a carbohydrate food literally begins in the mind. It's the body's way of getting a head start on digesting your meal before the food even passes your lips.[4]

So think about the typical dieter who denies herself nourishing or satisfying food, who doesn't fulfill her CPDR requirement and therefore is constantly fantasizing about forbidden foods such as desserts and pastries. She'll be in a continuous cephalic phase insulin response and thus producing insulin even though there are no carbohydrates or sugar for that insulin to act upon. This means that insulin levels will be artificially high and the insulin will be sitting around with nothing to do. By default, this chemical will then perform its secondary function, which is to store fat and inhibit muscle growth. Add to this the stress of dieting and denying oneself food and satisfaction and our dieter will also produce more cortisol—yet another fat-storage hormone. So by constantly fantasizing about carbohydrate-rich foods and leading a stressful life, our dieter will have the exact pieces in place for chronically elevated insulin and cortisol—the precursors for "noncaloric" weight gain.

The point is not to stop fantasizing about waffles and ice cream. The point is that maybe you simply need to give yourself permission to eat it, be aware that you are eating it, get the satisfaction (the CPDR) your brain is requiring, and move on to the next life experience. If you get what you want you won't need to be constantly thinking about what you don't have. It's that simple.

For many people, satisfaction is a radical concept. We've been conditioned to believe that to lose weight we need to deny ourselves food, deny ourselves pleasure, and wage a war against our appetite with all the firepower we can muster. But by fighting the biology of the body, we create the very condition we so sincerely struggle to avoid. Checking in when we eat as opposed to checking out ignites metabolism and fulfills the body's inborn need to dine.

More Awareness, Less Weight

Lisa, a thirty-seven-year-old lawyer in a banking firm, came to see me to lose weight. As a single woman her job was her life and she worked long hours to prove it. Lisa was bubbly and outgoing; yet, as she confided to me, the eight pounds she gained several years back was driving her crazy. She wanted to fall in love and start a family, but being overweight was for her an unacceptable obstacle.

Lisa was frustrated because it seemed she was doing everything correct to lose weight, but she hadn't dropped a pound in two years. Her diet was as follows. She had a cup of coffee in the morning and either skipped breakfast altogether or ate a yogurt as she ran out the door. She also skipped lunch several days each week; when she did eat lunch she would have either a small salad or half of a turkey sandwich. By three o'clock in the afternoon she was always ravenous and usually had a headache. At this point she'd have some chips, cookies, or candy and a diet soda. She'd finish work by seven o'clock, exercise hard at the gym for an hour, and would start dinner around eight thirty or nine o'clock. This was usually a small portion of Chinese or Italian take-out eaten in front of the TV. Several hours after dinner she'd be hungry again and would snack on popcorn, chips, or frozen yogurt until bedtime.

So here she was, eating a small amount of total calories and exercising hard each day, and she was still eight pounds overweight. She felt that her dinner and the snack after it was her only "downfall," but she was so hungry in the evening that she couldn't possibly eat less. She thought that perhaps she had a willpower problem that I could help her with, some magic trick to take away her hunger in the after-work hours.

I asked Lisa if she was a fast eater, a moderate eater, or a slow eater. She replied "very fast." I then asked if she liked food. She replied with childlike animation that she absolutely loved food. As you might imagine, my next question to Lisa was this: "If you love food so much, why don't you eat real food and have a real meal? Why do you rush through every eating experience? Why would you shovel food down in front of the TV? Wouldn't you want to make sure that if something truly gave you satisfaction, it would last long and you would completely savor the experience?"

I suggested that even though her food choices weren't the best, the root of Lisa's problem was not with nutrition per se but with awareness. Lisa was "out to lunch" whenever she ate. And that lack of awareness was what enabled her to eat a diet severely lacking in quality. She thought her downfall was in the evening time when she couldn't stop herself from eating. Her true downfall, though, was during the day. By skipping meals, eating too few calories, being deprived of micronutrients (vitamins, minerals) and macronutrients (proteins, fats), and having a boring diet, Lisa was setting herself up for nighttime binge eating. She hadn't fulfilled her cephalic phase requirements—the need for taste, pleasure, and awareness—during breakfast and lunch. Her brain was interpreting this nutrient deprivation and awareness deprivation as hunger. Finally, in the evening Lisa could no longer fight the natural, healthy, inborn urge to eat. That's when her "resistance" broke down and the floodgates opened. Her body cried out for whatever it could find to make up for its lack of nourishment.

Can you see how Lisa's intense need to eat at night was her body's attempt to correct an earlier imbalance? Unfortunately, when she finally had a significant meal, she did so at rapid-fire speed in front of the TV, which caused a further lack of cephalic phase fulfillment and the desire for yet another "meal"—a continuous snack—soon after her dinner.

The remedy I proposed to Lisa was to eat every meal and snack with awareness. No more skipping meals. Improve the quality of what she ate. Have a more robust breakfast and lunch, which meant including quality protein and fat such as eggs, fish, nut butters, salads with beans or tofu or quality meats. Slow down. Pretend the race is over and you are relaxing at the finish line. Kill the TV during dinner. Light a candle, play some music, invite a friend over, and feel nourished by food.

Lisa looked at me as if I were asking her to strip naked and dance in front of her family. But here's what she said about what happened from following those suggestions.

"I thought my biggest challenge would be to eat more food and enjoy it because I'm totally conscious about calories and fat grams. In fact, it was much harder for me to pay attention with food. I realized that I'm pretty much ADD when it comes to eating. I really wanted to believe that this would all work, because what I was doing certainly wasn't working. It didn't take long for me to discover, for the first time, a place of calm inside myself with food, a calm I had no idea existed."

By eating with awareness and fulfilling her CPDR, Lisa wasn't ravenous anymore at three o' clock or after dinner. She didn't need more willpower; she just needed more attention. Because she wasn't nutrient deprived or starving herself during the day, Lisa's headaches quickly disappeared. She was eating more calories along with more healthy fat, and she was happier. Within five weeks, Lisa lost exactly eight pounds. Focusing on nutrition changes alone would never have taken Lisa where she wanted to go. Awareness was the key to her breakthrough.

The Brain in Your Belly

Thus far we've looked at awareness as it's experienced in the brain. But there's another kind of intelligence that's an equally potent metabolic force, and it's found in the belly. Have you ever had "butterflies" in your stomach? A "lump" in your throat? Have you ever been moved by a strong and undeniable "gut feeling" about something or someone? Few people would say they had an elbow feeling or a kidney feeling, but gut feelings are highly regarded as a source of intuitive knowing and insight in many cultures around the globe. As it turns out, gut thoughts and feelings are not a fanciful notion but a physiological fact. Rather than the one brain found in our head, scientists have revealed that we have two brains—the other one is located in the digestive tract.

Known as the enteric nervous system (ENS), the gut's brain is housed under the mucosal lining and between the muscular layers of the esophagus, the stomach, and the small and large intestines. The enteric nervous system is a rich and complicated network of neurons and neurochemicals that sense and control events in the digestive tract and, remarkably, can sense and respond to events in other parts of the body, including the brain. Amazingly, when scientists finally counted the number of nerve cells in the gut-brain, they found it contained over one hundred million neurons—more than the number of nerve cells in the spinal cord.[5] What's fascinating to note is that researchers have observed a significantly greater flow of neural traffic from the ENS to the head-brain than from the head-brain to the ENS.[6] In other words, rather than the head informing the digestive system what to eat and how to metabolize, the locus of command is stationed in the belly.

In addition to an extensive network of neurons, the entire digestive tract is also lined with cells that produce and receive a variety of neuropeptides and neurochemicals, the same substances, in fact, that were previously thought to be found in the brain alone. These include serotonin, dopamine, norepinephrine, and glutamate. Even more eye-opening is that many hormones and chemicals previously thought to exist only in the gut were later found to be active in the brain. These include insulin, cholecystokinin, vasoactive intestinal protein, motilin, gastrin, somatostatin, thyrotropin releasing hormone, neurotensin, secretin, substance P, glucagon, and bombesin.[7]

The enteric nervous system (the gut-brain) and the central nervous system (the head-brain) also share another intriguing similarity. In the sleep state, the head-brain moves through cycles of ninety minutes of slow-wave sleep frequencies, immediately followed by rapid eye movement (REM) sleep in which dreams are produced. The gut-brain also moves through a nightly cycle of ninety minutes of slow-wave muscular contractions followed by brief spurts of rapid muscular movements. Is your gut dreaming?

Another compelling discovery is that the entire digestive tract is lined with specialized cells that produce and receive endorphins and enkephalins, chemicals that yield an array of sensations including joy, satisfaction, and pain relief. Most of the digestive sensations we are aware of tend to be negative ones, such as digestive upset and discomfort. Yet the warm gut feelings we sometimes experience after a satisfying meal or an exciting encounter are, in part, the enteric nervous system squirting pleasure chemicals at distant and neighboring cells.

As many of us know, the gut is often a barometer of our emotional states and stresses. Those who suffer from peptic ulcer, irritable bowel syndrome, heartburn, upset stomach, and other conditions would certainly concur. So when we say we can't "stomach" a situation or something makes us want to "gag," we are expressing real-life psycho-physiological sensations that arise from the enteric nervous system—the brain in the belly. Perhaps this is why the gut produces an abundance of a class of chemicals known as the benzodiazepines. These psychoactive substances are the active ingredients in the prescription drugs Valium and Xanax.[8] That's right, your gut naturally produces these drugs, in their exact chemical form, without a prescription and at no extra cost.

In Japan, the midsection is considered the seat of wisdom and the locus of our center of gravity, both physical and spiritual. Known as the *hara,* this place of ultimate balance is centered around a point just below the navel. The Japanese quite literally refer to the hara as their place of higher thought just as Americans would point to the head as the location of "central command." In other words, when we Americans say in a convincing tone "I know," we'll point to our heads. When the Japanese say "I know," they point to the belly. That's because the Japanese are, in part, accessing the neurochemical potential of the gut-brain. Americans express this understanding to a different degree when they compliment someone by saying, "You've got guts." Seldom do we praise others for having a liver or a spleen.

What all this means is that there's a tremendous amount of brain power in your belly, and such power goes largely untapped. You've probably heard the estimates that we use less than 10 percent of our brain capacity. Well, the same applies for our use of the gut-brain's potential.

So if you think you have a problem because your brain can't process all the contradictory information about diet fed to you by the media and the experts, think again. You really don't have a problem. Your brain isn't equipped to handle all that input by itself. It's not designed to handle a "high-fact" diet. When it comes to food, we are physiologically wired to hear the gut-brain speak its mind. The head-brain plays a supportive role.

Seldom will you see a lion all confused and anxious about which would be the best nutritional choice for the evening meal—zebra or caribou—or whether hippopotamus should be avoided altogether because it's too high in fat. Animals instinctively know what to eat. So do we. We just don't know that we know this.

Usually when people decide to focus on the belly it's about making the belly tighter or tougher. But let's take care of first things first. Make the belly smarter before endeavoring to make it harder. The less intelligent your gut, the more difficult it will be for your belly to find its proper tone. A well-defined muscle is an intelligent one. The obsession that so many Americans have with "tight abs" is a misplaced desire to use the wisdom of the midsection more proficiently. By having "the guts" to trust our ability to access gut-knowing, ego-driven fears naturally fall away and our true self-respect is revealed.

Week 3: Your Primary Task

This week is your opportunity to reap the metabolic rewards of awareness. Your primary task is to be present with food and to access the enteric nervous system—the seat of your gut wisdom. You'll learn to use relaxed awareness and the brain-in-the-belly to help determine which foods to eat and in what amounts.

Exercise: Be Awake at the Plate

This is your most fundamental exercise for the week: At each meal and every snack, choose to be present.

Notice your food. See it, touch it, and taste it with presence. Connect with it. Stay awake to your surroundings. Absorb all the nutrients of your meal—the colors and textures, the people with whom you're eating and your conversations, all the ambiance and nuances of the eating experience. If you find yourself thinking about the past or plotting your future, let it go. If you're off in some fantasy land, come back to Earth and be nice to your food. Allow yourself to be gently alert no matter what you eat, where you eat, or whom you're eating with. Notice the times when you go on automatic pilot while eating. In these moments simply remind yourself to wake up.

Even if you're eating something "forbidden" or bingeing on ice cream, your task is still to eat with awareness. That's because the more present you are at such times and the more you savor the experience, the sooner you'll satisfy your CPDR requirement and the less you'll need to eat. If you habitually watch TV or read while you eat, try going on a media-free diet for the week and note the difference in your body. If you constantly eat on the move, sit down and settle in with your food. Hopefully you'll find that being aware is not some nuisance diet strategy, nor is it a form of constraint or punishment. It feels good. It's personally satisfying. And the fact is, it's metabolically inspiring.

During this week it might be helpful to ask yourself "Why would I choose to be unaware? What is it that would influence me to go unconscious when I eat?" Sometimes we check out because we want to escape reality—usually an uncomfortable feeling or event. For many of us, though, eating without awareness is a habit we learned from a culture that has a love affair with speed. Chances are after your one-week experiment in aware eating a new habit will emerge. You'll naturally remind yourself to be awake at the plate.

Exercise: Gut Wisdom Inventory

As we get older the brain actually gets smarter. It has more life experience, information, and wisdom to pull from. It is the same with the gut-brain. Throughout your years your gut-brain accumulates a tremendous amount of data about what works and what doesn't. It knows your nutrient and food needs. It understands what gives you energy and what drains it. It identifies the ingredients you're sensitive and allergic to. It remembers how far you can push yourself with poor-quality foods. It realizes how much is too much. It determines the amount of alcohol, sugar, and caffeine you can honestly handle. It's recorded every meal that served you well and those that didn't. The gut-brain is your built-in nutrition sage.

With this in mind, take an inventory of all the important and pertinent lessons your gut-brain has learned about eating and nutrition throughout your life. Be specific, and make your list as complete as possible. Which foods make you feel best? Which ones pull you down?

Are there foods that once worked fine but are now hard to tolerate? Are there "forbidden" foods you just can't live without? What times during the day are best for you to eat? Which combinations of food upset your digestion? What foods do you know your body wants more of? You can think of this exercise as the writing of the nutrition-instruction booklet for your body.

As you consider what to include, take some deep breaths into your belly. Relax your mind and ask your gut to do the talking. Empower the brain in your belly to speak, and honor the wisdom of your lifelong experience.

When finished, reread and absorb the wisdom and information you've revealed to yourself. Do any entries stand out? Are there any new insights about you and your metabolism? Any particular nutrition truths for your body that you need to remind yourself of more consistently?

The first practical step necessary for tapping into ENS intelligence is to breathe into the belly. In the yoga tradition there's a saying that has helped practitioners reach for greater levels of mastery in working with the body: "Where attention goes, energy flows." Decades of research in biofeedback has certainly proved this axiom, for when we focus on most any area of the body we can increase blood flow, alter bioelectric potential, and influence the secretion of numerous biochemicals. Breathing into the belly increases its oxygen uptake and activates the ENS. It makes the gut function smarter. Think about it: an oxygen deficit can cause damage to the head-brain while a surplus yields improvements in memory, performance, and creativity. The same holds true for the gut-brain. Deprive it of oxygen and the enteric nervous system goes sluggish. It can require more food to register sensations of pleasure, satisfaction, and fullness. Flood the belly with oxygen and the gut-brain is responsive and alert.

Once you're centered in breathing, your next step is simple: ask the brain in your belly for advice. Silently question the ENS: "Is this a good food for me to eat right now?" or "What meal would be best for my body at this time?" or "What amount of this food is best in this moment?" Allow your mind to be silent and let the answers emerge

Access Gut Wisdom

A Japanese billionaire once remarked that his simple formula for success was this. Before he proceeds with any deal or project, he first "swallows" it to see how it digests. If what he swallows metabolizes smoothly, the deal is made. But with any hint of indigestion negotiations are ended. This may sound to you and me like a superstitious way to do business, but it's a telling example of how the genius of the ENS can be harnessed.

Learning to use your gut-brain is no different than discovering new ways to use your head-brain's innate capacity. It takes time, focus, and some trial and error. For many of us, ailments such as indigestion, bloating, heartburn, and gas aren't so much digestive problems as they are awareness problems—a lack of attention to the ongoing feedback available to us from the ENS.

It's time to use all our "smarts" when it comes to nutrition and health. The key to accessing the abundant intelligence of the ENS is respect. Allow for the possibility that your gut-brain can be a most trusted advisor. Honor the cosmic design within you, the built-in sage that exists to teach you about how to absorb and assimilate the world. Slow down and listen closely to the messages that await you, the genius that resides in your core.

from your gut's insightful source. Some people describe light, intuitive sensations that inform them whether or not to choose a particular food. Others receive clear and unmistakable feedback from their ENS that sounds like a resounding "yes" or "no" answer. Before you actually "down" a food or choose your meal, symbolically swallow it and experience the results. See what kind of gut feelings arise.

If you're concerned that you'll ask your ENS what to eat and you'll get the wrong answer, don't worry. You've been wrong once or twice before in life and you're still here. This is training. You may be thinking: "But what if I ask my gut-brain and it tells me to eat lots of chocolate?" In such cases, you may need to override suspicious instructions and try to determine which brain was really doing the talking. Or you may wish to simply comply and note the results. Trial and error is how evolution works. Learn to be responsible, and learn to trust yourself. Personal empowerment equals metabolic empowerment.

To summarize:

1. Before any meal or snack, sit comfortably and take five deep breaths into your midsection.
2. Let the breath flow in and out naturally and generously without holding or forcing it. Feel what a fully oxygenated gut feels like.
3. Consciously rest your mind and ask for insights from the wisdom of your ENS. Silently inquire: "What foods would best nourish me at this time?" "Is this particular food a good choice?" "Is this a good combination of food choices?"
4. Let the answers arise effortlessly, with a quiet mind and without censorship.
5. Follow the directions of your gut's wisdom and note the results.

Remember, you're tapping into a center of intelligence that most of us are unaccustomed to using. Like learning a foreign language or a new style of dance, expect to feel a little awkward and uncertain. Mistakes are really learning experiences in disguise. The more you call upon your ENS intelligence, the smarter it becomes. Consider this a lifelong practice in which your gut-brain will become a primary consultant in all your nutrition affairs. So, no matter what the experts are saying and how confusing their advice, you'll always have your own expert to call upon for the final word. This is what we do anyway. Some part of us decides who we'll listen to. By accessing gut wisdom, we learn to make deliberate, empowered, and deeply informed choices.

Another version of this technique is to ask the ENS for feedback. Once you've taken a bite of a particular food or dish, ask the gut "How does that feel? Did this food work for me?" After a meal ask yourself: "Is there a correlation between what I ate then and how I feel now?" Many people report that asking for feedback gives nutritional information and insights that are highly specific. For example, some of us eat certain combinations of foods that irritate digestion and suppress metabolism, but we don't know it until we listen for feedback. There are plenty of helpful books on food combining that tell you what to eat, but in my experience, each of us is metabolically unique. You have your own food-combining system that, ultimately, only you can discover.

Exercise: Eating to the Point of Energy

Most people eat until they're filled with food. Whenever this occurs, we must generate more metabolic force to process such a big meal. More metabolic force means an increased amount of oxygen and blood must be sent to the digestive organs. This extra blood flow will be pulled from our extremities—our arms and legs and, to a small degree, our head. And what happens when we pull some blood flow from the head? We feel tired and sluggish. Eating until we're full can also lead to digestive upset, heartburn, stress-induced digestive shutdown, and impaired nutrient metabolism. So instead of eating to the point where you're filled with food, eat to the point you're filled with energy.

The yogis of ancient India described a special point in any meal whereupon, if you stopped eating at that time, you'd walk away from the table with more *prana*—more energy or life force—than when you sat down. Finding this "point of energy" takes some experimentation, but you'll certainly be well-rewarded for proving its existence to yourself.

This technique requires that we check in with gut wisdom throughout the meal. Ask the ENS: "How do I feel? How is my energy level? Do I still feel light? Am I starting to feel heavy?" Estimate the point at which you feel filled with energy yet not filled with food. Your belly will feel light; you'll feel slightly "up"; you will still be a little hungry yet you'll translate that hunger and desire for more food into the next thing you do after your meal.

Conversely, when you eat even one bite past the point of energy you'll start to feel heavier.

Remember, you're asking these questions of your gut, not your head. The more you engage your ENS, the more it learns. The key is to simply be interested enough in what your gut-brain can tell you. As you move through a week's worth of meals, you'll get better at instinctively finding your point of energy. The reward will be a feeling of energized lightness and a sense of satisfaction that you worked smarter, not harder, to nourish yourself in a good way. Your focus is not to limit calories, even though decreased intake may certainly result. Your focus is to access gut wisdom and be guided by it.

This technique is especially useful if you know you'll need all of your brain power at a certain time of the day—for example, for a meeting, a negotiation, or a test. In short, the meal just before this time should be a light one. That will ensure more blood flow to your brain and make you smarter and more alert. Conversely, if you're in a business negotiation and you want the upper hand, spread a huge and delicious buffet before your unsuspecting associates. They'll be so appreciative.

To summarize:

1. Set the intention at the beginning of your meal to eat to the point of energy.
2. Observe your energy level at least four times as you eat. Your energy level means your sense of vibrancy, lightness, and alertness.
3. Observe your satisfaction level as you eat.
4. Observe your satiation level as you eat.
5. Guesstimate the point at which you can leave the meal with more energy than when you started. You'll still be slightly hungry, you won't be totally satiated, you may feel like eating more, and you'll translate your "hunger" and "desire for more" into the next thing you do. You will know you've gone past the point of energy if you begin to feel heavy, sluggish, tired, dense, or unfocused.

Eating to the point of energy is a wonderful tool that will help liberate you from the confusion and fear that surrounds the question "How much should I eat?" For the majority of people, food measurements have become a source of disempowerment and an energy drain. How can we expect portioned sizes to work for us if we eat in a stress state, without awareness and satisfaction or with little oxygen from shallow breathing? As we've seen, the body will absolutely demand that we eat more under any of these circumstances, and its efficiency in digesting and calorie burning will suffer. If the simple act of controlling portions to lose weight was effective, we'd all listen and do it and it would have worked long ago. Something has been missing. Fortify your diet with vitamin A—awareness—and your power to metabolize will truly grow.

It's certainly worth noting how the majority of diet and nutrition books on the market have us counting protein grams, fat grams, carbohydrate grams, portions, calories, servings, and points. You'd think we were consuming a bunch of numbers. It's as if eating is a sporting event where you keep score or a business transaction with the body where we track debits and credits. We are truly "crunching the numbers."

Of course, counting in such a manner certainly has its place for some, but for most of us it's time to graduate to a new level of freedom. Visit any culture on planet Earth where a traditional or quality diet is eaten—regions in Asia, Europe, Central America, Australia, New Zealand, Iceland, and the Pacific Rim—and you'll find people who are lean, healthy, happy about their bodies, and thoroughly bemused by the concept of calorie counting.

It's time we learned from the real experts. Give up all numbers. Let go of counting anything you eat. Live. Eat. Believe in yourself. Find your natural intelligence. Trust it. Respect it. Honor the beautiful nourishment process that we live inside and that lives within us. Embrace the vivaciousness, the succulence, and the naturalness of eating. You and I have an instinctive and effortless appetite that will clearly speak to us when we let go of fear and listen. Make the leap.

🐌 Key Lessons

- The cephalic phase digestive response (CPDR) is proof positive that our awareness of a meal greatly impacts its nutritional value.

- For optimum nutritional metabolism—when you eat, eat.

- The less aware we are of a meal as we eat, the more the brain will signal us to consume excess food.

- The enteric nervous system (ENS) is a separate yet interconnected brain in the digestive tract.

- The ENS holds a vast amount of wisdom and information about our nutritional and metabolic needs.

- We can access ENS—gut wisdom—through mind/body awareness to determine the foods and their amounts that will best serve us.

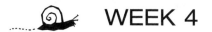 **WEEK 4**

The Metabolic Power of Rhythm

The moon invented natural rhythm.
Civilization uninvented it.

TOM ROBBINS

Rhythm is everywhere. Each particle of our being moves and pulsates, dances and sings, and keeps to the beat of a brilliantly conceived symphony. The whole of our biology is a fantastic clockwork of precise chemical and hormonal rhythms whose timing is critical for our survival and well-being. Your heart beating is a rhythm. Your lungs breathing, inhaling and exhaling vital atmosphere, is a rhythm. The electrochemical pulsation of the brain is a rhythm. So is the menstrual cycle, waking and sleeping, digesting and eliminating, and the contraction and expansion of every cell, vessel, and organ in the body. Interfere with any of these and disease or death shall follow.

Master rhythm and you master metabolism.

Indeed, much of what ails us from a nutritional perspective—weight gain, fatigue, digestive complaints, carbohydrate craving, overeating—can be resolved by entraining with the kinds of rhythms that naturally and effortlessly regenerate us. Let's take a look at how we can better understand and harness this important metabolic force.

Hot Rhythms

One of the simplest and most reliable ways to measure the metabolic rate of the human body is to take its temperature. The hotter you are, the more metabolic you'll be. Recall that the Latin name for our midsection—solar plexus—means "gathering place for the sun." This highlights how long we've known that the basic design of the human form is a capturing device for the sun's energy. The more efficiently we harness the sun's warmth, the better we digest, assimilate, and calorie burn.

It's no accident that we use temperature metaphors to describe what excites us. An energetic person is called "a fireball," an attractive person is "hot," we "warm up" to some people while others leave us "cold."

As evolutionary fate would have it, body temperature has a rhythm that is consistent and predictable for most everyone, and this daily rhythmic fluctuation reveals some important insights into unleashing our metabolic potential.[1] During the evening and early morning hours when we sleep, body temperature drops. It makes sense that our bodies are cooler at this time because we're not busy hunting for animals in the jungle or hunting for bargains at the mall. Our muscles have little work to do at this time; the body is in a state of rest, healing, and repair of all its tissues. We do burn calories as we sleep, but not even close to the amount we use up in our waking hours. As we sleep, the body is in a fasting state—assuming we didn't eat a big meal just before bed.

The moment your eyes open in the morning, body temperature automatically begins to rise. This is the same thing as saying your metabolism wakes up when you do. It makes biological sense because now the sun is up: it's time to find food, find a mate, do battle, and perhaps do a few good deeds. Even if you stayed in bed all day and didn't move, your temperature/metabolism would still elevate because we're programmed to entrain with the rhythms of the sun.

Because you're naturally heating up in the morning, eating at this time is a smart bet if you're trying to lose weight. Adding food to your gut will increase metabolic rate even more and provide your body with the nutrients it's already preparing to process. Think of your gut as a furnace. When you add fuel, the heat rises.

There are, of course, exceptions to every nutritional rule. Many people who live in hot-weather climates do great on no breakfast, a light breakfast, or a fruit breakfast. You'll also find that you might do well on a substantial breakfast in the colder months but will be drawn to eat lighter in the early hours during the warmer seasons. You may also go through periods where the first meal you eat isn't until lunch, and that too works fine, until your metabolism shifts into its next phase.

Body temperature continues a slow, steady rise and subsequently peaks around noon. It will exactly reach its apex the very moment the sun finds its high point in the sky—this is a little known scientific fact that shows our profound connection to the cosmos. Our digestive force is therefore hottest at lunchtime. It makes sense, then, that our largest meal would be best consumed at this time, when our ability to pulverize food is strongest.

After our metabolic peak at high noon, body temperature dips for the period between approximately two o'clock and five o'clock in the afternoon. It shouldn't surprise you that just as we feel more awake when body temperature is rising, we feel sleepy when it's falling. So if you've ever felt that there's something wrong with you because your energy drops somewhere between 2-ish and 5-ish, don't worry—you're perfectly normal. Most people you ask will tell you that they feel tired during this time. It's the human rhythm. Lions love to lounge around and absorb after their big kill. So do you and I.

Body energy—metabolism—in the form of blood flow and oxygenation is rerouted to digestion after our midday meal. The result is that we feel tired. The people in many European and Latin American countries typically have their biggest meal at lunchtime—the peak metabolic time slot of digestion and calorie burning. Then they take a siesta. Businesses shut down, social activity goes quiet, and people snooze. They are honoring and working with the natural rhythms of the body.

Entire cultures are designed to function in relation to digestive rhythms.

Except ours.

In America, most of us tank up on caffeine or sugar in the metabolic decline of 2:00 to 5:00 PM, pushing through our fatigue in service to a way of life that values the overdrive gear more than any other speed. Can you imagine what life would be like if you could relax during this time and let go of achieving and conquering? Numerous studies have shown that one or two fifteen- to twenty-minute rest periods during the day will profoundly increase cognitive function, physical performance, mood, and energy. You don't even need to sleep during this time. It's simply about rest, stillness, closing off outside sensations, and recharging your batteries.

Simply put, resting is a metabolic enhancer.

At around 4:00 to 6:00 PM body temperature starts to rise again. This is when most people feel their energy return. It's also when the English stop for tea time. It makes perfect sense to do your caffeine at this point, when metabolism is picking up anyway. By around nine o'clock, body temperature begins another downward trend in preparation for sleep. Indeed, sleep research reveals that we cannot fall asleep soundly unless temperature is dropping. Anything, then, that would raise body heat in the late evening would be counterproductive to good sleep. Recall that the act of eating raises body temperature. A big meal before bed would therefore interfere with your slumber. Once again, though, Americans have it backward. We tend to do a small to nonexistent breakfast, a moderate-size lunch, and more often than not a big dinner before bed. And this is exactly what you ought to do if your goal is restless sleep and weight gain.

It's About Time

As every musician, scientist, and mechanic knows, rhythm is measured in quantity per unit of time. Your heart rate is counted in number of beats per minute. The speed at which you drive your car is measured in miles per hour. And though no official calculation exists for how well you metabolize and burn calories at different times of the day, I can assure you of this—metabolism, too, is all about time.

When you eat is as important as what you eat.

In a typical study, researchers put a group of people on a 2,000 calorie diet. In the first part of the study test subjects could only eat their 2,000 calories at breakfast. They ate nothing else for the rest of the day. With this one meal in the morning, everyone either lost weight or maintained their existing weight. In the second phase of the study, the same exact people ate the same exact 2,000 calorie diet, except this time they could only eat it at dinner. With this one meal for the entire day, eaten in the evening, every single person in the study gained weight.[2]

Can you see why counting calories to lose weight can be a waste of energy?

Timing is everything. Sumo wrestlers have known for centuries that large meals eaten in the late evening hours will give them the physical advantage they covet most—flab. Simply put, we calorie burn less efficiently in the evening hours.

An important aspect of metabolism that popular science tends to overlook is the fact that exercising your digestive function, especially at the right time, makes metabolism stronger. Nutritional value is given not just in the vitamins and nutrients in our food but is generated by the process that the body goes through to pulverize, digest, assimilate, and eliminate a meal. Eating is like an exercise, and food is the weight your body must "lift" to build its metabolic strength. When we consistently fail to give the gastrointestinal tract its proper workout, it loses its tone and we grow metabolically weak.

If you wanted to optimize the benefits of exercise you wouldn't do your workout at the time of day when you were most tired. Likewise, if you want to get the ultimate metabolic benefit of eating, don't eat your most substantial and nutrient-dense meal when your digestion is on a downturn—the evening hours. Unless you're seriously considering an unusual career change, I suggest you relinquish the Sumo diet immediately. Eating little food during the day and much in the evening will never take you where you want to go when it comes to optimizing energy and burning calories.

The First Meal Sets the Rhythm

Let's say that you wake up in the morning and decide not to eat breakfast. You figure "Well, I'm not hungry, I'll just have some coffee, maybe a little bit of cereal or a muffin or a bagel. If I eat this meager amount of food until lunch I'll be a good girl and lose weight."

Bad girl.

Body temperature is naturally rising in the morning to prepare you for a metabolic resurgence. In the absence of food, or in the absence of enough food, the body gets concerned. It says something like: "Hey, I thought I was preparing to raise metabolism with a morning meal. I thought my food source was abundant and dependable. There's nothing here. I must be shipwrecked on a desert island. Or maybe there's a famine. Better slow down metabolism—store fat and don't build any muscle because there are lean times ahead."

This genetically programmed survival response is a brilliant mechanism for supporting the continuation of life in times of emergency. When the brain senses trouble with the food supply, it does the most simple and impactful metabolic reprogramming to conserve energy—store fat and forget about building muscle. Just the opposite of what you're trying to do by denying yourself food.

To make matters worse for weight loss, many people have a breakfast that consists of one ingredient: coffee. Coffee by itself raises cortisol levels.[3] The coffee lobby doesn't want you to know this (I used to work for them) because this basically means that coffee can chemically mimic the stress response and cause abdominal weight gain. This doesn't mean coffee is bad. It just means that when you combine lack of food (survival response—elevated cortisol), anxiety (stress response—elevated cortisol), and caffeine (mimics stress response—elevated cortisol), you have three factors that powerfully synergize to send cortisol production through the roof, suppressing digestive metabolism and depositing weight.

Again and again, we see the importance of cortisol levels in health and weight. Cortisol isn't a bad chemical. It's an integral component of an alive human body. Without it we couldn't exist. In the right quantities it helps maintain the proper functioning of every major system in the body. When we overproduce cortisol, though, we age prematurely, wear down our weakest links, and gain weight around the middle.

Strangely enough, the chemicals that wreak the most havoc in our lives and prove to be the most toxic are the ones we self-produce. That's why the biggest pharmaceutical companies in the world are busy behind the scenes perfecting home-test kits so you can measure your own cortisol levels. Of course, if you find that your cortisol level is too high, you can buy whatever drug they concoct to lower it. But you needn't wait for the next magic bullet to improve metabolism and lower your weight. No drug has ever worked for this purpose and none of them ever will. Just follow the inborn rhythms of the body and you'll liberate yourself while putting the diet-pill pushers out of business forever.

Now, let's imagine it's lunchtime. You've had your small or nonexistent breakfast and perhaps a second cup of coffee in the midmorning. You have some energy and you don't feel the need or the desire for a big lunch. Maybe you think you're being good by holding back on the calories; perhaps you don't have much time for lunch anyway, so why not grab half a sandwich, or a salad with a no-oil dressing, or have a late lunch at two or three o'clock?

If this is your strategy, what seems to be sensible is actually working against you. First, the body is designed to optimally digest and calorie burn when the sun is at its apex in the sky. By not putting fuel in the furnace at this time, or simply by not eating enough, you miss your peak metabolic window of opportunity, which is approximately 12:00 to 1:30 in the afternoon. Missing this opportunity is the equivalent of being all dressed up with no place to go. Chances are you'll be ravenous by three or four o'clock, maybe headachy or irritable, and grab an unhealthy snack. In other words, you'll be suffering from arrhythmia—being out of sync with your natural circadian flow.

And by eating a tiny breakfast and a minimal or late lunch, you assure major hunger in the evening. Many people who follow this arrhythmic sequence of events find that they have a substantial snack before dinner because they're so hungry they can't wait for the actual meal, or they're simply ravenous in the evening and eat a huge dinner, Sumo style.

The Metabolic Gift of Sleep

One of the downsides of consuming a high volume of food before bed is that we miss some of the great metabolic gifts of sleep. As you slumber at night the body shifts the bulk of its metabolic focus to maintenance, detoxification, repair, and growth of its tissues and organs. When you grow new muscle and bone, you do so as you sleep. The liver, which is our primary organ of detoxification, does the bulk of its work in the late evening and early morning hours. Sleep is not the most well publicized of our metabolic activators, nor is it the sexiest, but if this rhythm isn't fully honored we pay the price.

By consuming a big meal right before bed, much of the metabolic energy that is usually spent on maintenance, detoxification, repair, and growth is necessarily rerouted into digestion. That's simply how the body works. Short-term survival needs take precedence over long-term ones. So with an excess of blood flow and metabolism focused on processing your meal as you sleep, you'll most likely wake up feeling congested and heavy because you didn't detoxify fully during the night. The period between dinner and breakfast is evolution's built-in fast. That's because the fasting state is the ideal biological milieu to rebuild the body. And that's also why breakfast is called "break-fast"—we're ending this necessary period with food in the morning.

So if you wake up feeling tired and toxic from eating a large, late dinner because you didn't have real relaxed meals during the day, you'll naturally repeat this arrhythmic pattern. You won't be hungry in the morning because your body will still be in detoxification mode when instead it should be readying itself for the metabolically stimulating activity of eating. Lunch will then feel to your body like breakfast and dinner will be interpreted by your body as lunch—time for the biggest meal. Some time after the dinner that your body thought was lunch, you'll be looking for "dinner" and end up having late-night snacks.

Oftentimes you'll hear nutritionists recommend that you eat your evening meal about four hours before bedtime. A four-hour time period is sufficient for most people to metabolize a meal. You will then go to bed without raising your body temperature through the metabolic effect of food, thus increasing your probability of restful sleep. You'll also do what you were meant to do while lying in bed—healing, detoxifying, rebuilding, and so forth—without sidetracking vital metabolic force into digestion.

To accomplish this, you may need to retrain your body and reorient your lifestyle. Focus on having a smaller and earlier dinner and have a more robust breakfast. Eating a relaxed, sane, sensuous lunch makes it easier to have a lighter dinner. If you know you're going to have a late dinner and that's simply what your schedule is going to be because there's no way around it, you can still help yourself with this reliable trick: have a substantial snack sometime before dinner, approximately two to three hours earlier, and eat less at dinner. The snack will decrease your evening-time appetite and you'll essentially be buying these calories from dinner and expending them earlier, when you'll better use them and burn them anyway. This strategy is also useful if you find yourself coming home from work and feeling ravenous at dinner. By a substantial snack, I mean anything that has some healthy protein or fat: nuts and seeds, trail mix, peanut butter or almond butter with crackers or fruit, yogurt, hummus, guacamole, or bean dip.

Because of our work style, many of us ignore food and nourishment while we attend, frantically, to business. But this always catches up with us. The minute we return home from the office, the brain finally has permission to attend to our needs. But instead of calmly informing us that we neglected to rhythmically feed the body and nourish the soul during our workday, it jumps all over us like a neglected dog and barks out "I'm hungry!" The ravenous sensations we experience can be overwhelming, causing us to overeat. We then feel guilty and try to make up for our lack of willpower and control by following a tougher exercise regime.

Can you see how oftentimes our solutions to nutritional problems really have nothing to do with the actual problem? Is it clear how we can punish ourselves for all the wrong reasons when it comes to eating and exercise?

By planning a late-afternoon snack, then, you're making a preemptive strike against ravenous, out-of-control, after-work eating. You'll be making a conscious choice to attend to your universal right to nourish yourself, thereby short-circuiting the habit of denying yourself food and then devouring it. You'll also be making a powerful statement that your job doesn't supercede your health.

A Rhythmic Success Story

Peter, a fifty-two-year-old business consultant, spends time between New York, London, and Florida. With family and business in each of these locations, Peter leads a lifestyle that includes periods of intense travel and work interspersed with downtime that can last for several months. His reasons for seeing me were chronic bloating after meals, weight gain around the midsection, carbohydrate craving, and fatigue. Peter is a self-motivated man, so he was always exploring different ways to fix his symptoms—supplements, colon-cleansing programs, low-calorie diets, fruit-only breakfasts, and so on. He found success with all of these approaches but inevitably fell back into weight gain, fatigue, and bloating. He was tired of bouncing back and forth; he couldn't understand why everything initially worked yet ultimately failed, and he was tired of feeling tired.

When I asked Peter about his diet an interesting picture emerged. Breakfast was erratic. He either ate it or he didn't. If he did, breakfast was a croissant and coffee. Lunch went the same way—sometimes he ate it, sometimes he skipped it. He usually had a coffee if he missed lunch, and he might have a salad later on in the afternoon, or he would have some cheese or a candy bar. When he did eat lunch it was a turkey sandwich or pasta. He usually felt irritable and low mood in the midafternoon. Then he was ravenous by six o'clock. He'd have a huge dinner and would go to bed early feeling full and bloated. Remarkably, even when Peter wasn't working for weeks at a time, he still followed this erratic schedule even though he had plenty of space in his day to plan his meals.

Most nutritionists or doctors would use some fairly predictable strategies—low-calorie meal planning for weight loss, allergy testing or GI tests for bloating, and prescribing a long list of supplements or drugs for fatigue and depression. Indeed, Peter had been subjected to all these and more, and they were all sensible, well-chosen approaches. But nothing stuck. That's because Peter's core metabolic issue was never addressed. That issue was simply this: Peter had no rhythm.

He hadn't found a way to consistently and thoughtfully nourish himself. There was no coherence in how he cared for body and soul. Internally, he never made a commitment to true self-sustenance. He planned his finances but couldn't predict his next meal. He valued being busy but didn't know how to relax. He lived in fight-or-flight chemistry even when there was nothing chasing him or no one to attack. In that subtle biochemical state of inner fear and constant worrying, who has time for a thoughtful nutritional experience?

I suggested to Peter that the best dietary and medical strategies would never be of any use until he made the choice to abide by the law that every living creature is bound to—rhythm. Plan your breakfast, plan your lunch, plan your dinner and enjoy them as if each were your first meal on Earth, or your last. Either make the choice right now for nourishment to be a daily priority, or find another planet where stressful, haphazard meals of boring food make people happy and healthy.

The simple strategy of committing to rhythm had a profound effect. Peter stopped trying to fix his problem and began to create a daily rhythm that left little room for his problems to exist. He chose to start his day not by charging out of the gates in an urgent sprint but by slowly spreading his wings, embracing the world, and gently soaring. In other words, he created time to sit and eat a breakfast he enjoyed. He paid attention to his hunger in midmorning to see whether he needed a snack. He planned a celebrational lunch whenever he could. He brought food to work in case he needed a quality snack. And by the time he came to dinner it was no longer a "desperation meal" by which all his tension had to be resolved and all of his unfulfilled food desires had to be met. Dinner became a relaxed experience of light eating he looked forward to.

Rhythm is not about a mechanical timetable of feeding. It's about agreeing to be alive in a way that works. It's about respecting yourself enough to value the care of your body. It's about learning how to use vitamin T—time—so that metabolism is truly supported. When we live each day in stress chemistry, our cortisol level is constantly elevated. Not only does this chemical cause us to be more alert, it has an unusual added feature: cortisol skews our time perception. In other words, it has the pharmacological effect of making us feel as though we're behind schedule and time is running out. This, of course, is one of cortisol's ingenious functions because when the pack of wolves is after us, time really is running out. But when we self-generate this chemical day after day out of failing to relax, breathe, and be aware, we function as if the wolves are always there.

The key rhythm that Peter changed was an internal one, something found deep within that goes beyond the realm of nutrition and pills and meal planning. Peter accessed a quiet, secure place inside himself. Even though he was still the same guy with the same life, a part of him had finally stopped running. For so many years Peter had had an abundance of friends, family, and comforts but he hadn't fully learned to appreciate them. By slowing down and choosing life, Peter's world transformed. His digestive problems subsided within a few weeks and he had no more bloating or tiredness after meals. He was also happier about who he was. And within five months he lost twenty pounds.

Fortunately, though, Peter's problems didn't totally disappear, because every time he slipped back into a frenzied, fearful, arrhythmic lifestyle, his symptoms quickly returned. His digestive system became a barometer that alerted him about when he was falling off the wagon and into his old patterns of self-neglect. Peter didn't have a perfect relationship with health and weight, but he now had an authentic one.

Endless Summer

A final way we can work with rhythm to help transform weight and well-being is to change the eating habits that put us into a "prehibernation metabolism." Here's what I mean.

Our distant ancestors evolved an exquisite mechanism to take advantage of the abundance of food in the summer and the lack of it in the winter. They stayed up for the long daylight hours, loaded up on all the sweet fruits and berries they could find, and stored those foodstuffs as fat. Because winter is around the corner and lean times are ahead, it's best to eat as much as possible while the goodies are available. Evolution, therefore, figured out a way to stimulate our appetite to unusual lengths when the carbohydrates were available and to help us store them on our bodies. Again, insulin is the key substance we produce to accomplish this feat. Normally, insulin helps send carbohydrates in the form of sugar into our cells to provide us with energy. That's a good thing. When we consume an excess of carbohydrates, and the body accordingly produces too much insulin, we become insulin resistant; the body responds as if there's no insulin available and stores those carbs as body fat. That's also a good thing. You wouldn't want to keep sending sugar into the cells as you ate excessive amounts. Your cells would explode.

So as we evolved over eons of time, the chemistry of the body became radically different in the summertime as we prepared for colder months.[4] The availability of carbohydrate foods stimulated our hearty desire to consume them even more. By the time winter came, we'd be well-padded with body fat. We'd also have excess water weight from a high-carbohydrate diet, and our cholesterol level would be high because the body also turns carbohydrates into cholesterol to serve as an energy source and to plug up leaks in the cardiovascular system. Blood sugar level would be quite high (a diabetic state); sugar in the blood literally functions as an antifreeze for the cold months. If you tasted the antifreeze in your car, by the way, it would taste sweet.

We can observe this physiologic pattern in hibernating mammals. A bear loads up on fruit in the summer, gets fat, has high cholesterol and high blood pressure—basically, the bear is in a high–blood sugar diabetic state. And all these "diseases"—which are really helpful and necessary in the short term—are naturally resolved in the winter months as the bear burns its fat stores and its blood cholesterol, loses its water weight, sheds its diabetic antifreeze state, and comes out of hibernation looking svelte and feeling hungry and ready for action.

Now here's the problem: even though modern humans aren't attempting to fatten up in the summer, many of us consume sugar, candy, cookies, crackers, cake, pasta, bread, donuts, rice, potatoes, and wheat products in great quantity day in and day out throughout the year. And by doing so, our system goes into rhythmic meltdown. The body thinks it's in an endless summer; we are forever in a prehibernation state. Couple this with lack of sleep, excess exposure to artificial light, and increased stress, and fat storage is multiplied. So the sooner you stop preparing to hibernate, the better. This means eating less poor-quality carbohydrates and getting more sleep. I'm not saying staying up late is bad, nor am I saying that sugar or carbohydrates are bad. I'm just alerting you to the fact that if these features dominate your lifestyle, you won't come very close to your true metabolic potential.

So with all this information about the metabolic power of rhythm, the questions to ask yourself are these: Do I have rhythm? Is there a coherent flow to my day? Do I have a lifestyle with regular times for meals, rest, enjoyment, sleep, and nourishment? If the answer to these questions is no, then your first step is this.

Choose rhythm.

This means letting go of the shotgun approach to eating where you grab what you can, when you can and instead caring for yourself by making nourishment a consistent priority.

Here's how to get started.

Week 4: Your Primary Task

This week is your opportunity to reap the metabolic rewards of rhythm. Learn to use the key principles of rhythmic nutrition to your greatest advantage, and the benefits for body, mind, and soul will be immediate. Your primary task for week 4 is to incorporate these key rhythmic strategies into your life: eating regularly, balancing your macronutrients at meals, planning the time and size of your meals, planning your daily meals and snacks, using caffeine wisely, and getting regular rest and regular play.

Exercise: Eat Regularly

Begin your week with the foundational commitment to have regular and consistent meals. Make eating a predictable part of your daily flow. This is the key to unlocking the metabolic power of rhythm. No more skipping meals and no more fuzzy boundaries around eating—"I was too busy to have lunch," "I lost track of the time," "I stop for meals when I can squeeze it in." As best as you can, each evening plan your menus and your meal times for the next day. Know that you're going to have a breakfast, a lunch, and a dinner. Choose rhythm. Make your mealtimes important. Honestly look at your schedule and see what adjustments you need to make to create time for three solid eating experiences each day. Do you need to wake up a little earlier to have a sit-down breakfast? What needs to happen at home or work so you can have a regular lunch? How can you enlist the help of those around you? If you travel or have irregular work or parenting schedules, commit to thoughtful advanced meal planning. Take food with you when necessary.

Exercise: Balance Macronutrients at Meals

If you've tried unsuccessfully to lose weight or if you're experiencing fatigue, here are some excellent strategies that incorporate the use of macronutrients—protein, fat, and carbohydrate proportions. As best you can, eliminate "carbohydrate only" breakfasts. This means no morning meals that consist of only cereal, oatmeal, a donut, bagel, muffin, granola bar, croissants, toast with jam or margarine, and so forth. These foods are not necessarily bad. This is simply an experiment to see what happens to your metabolism with such a change.

This week, for each breakfast ask yourself: "Where's the healthy protein and fat?" Let these two macronutrients be at the center of your first meal of the day. Try to include one of these choices in your breakfast: organic peanut butter, almond butter, or other nut butters (with fruit or a slice of whole-grain toast); whole free-range eggs; full fat organic yogurt with some nuts and seeds; organic cottage cheese; fish or smoked fish; free-range turkey sausage; or high-quality cheese. Include a slice of quality whole-grain bread and/or fresh fruit as you desire. If you want cereal, use organic oatmeal and have it with some nuts and seeds or with nut butter or yogurt. Breakfast is not your time to count calories. Unless you eat ten pounds of cream cheese, your body will preferentially burn whatever you eat in the morning. That's a metabolic law.

Notice I'm not saying that you should be fanatic about eliminating carbohydrates. We're just making them a side dish when you want them, not the main course. As far as portions go, eat an amount that leaves you satisfied but not tired and full. Trust your choices.

For lunch, the same basic principles apply. Once again ask yourself: Where's the healthy protein and fat? As best you can, try having one of the following at the center of your lunch: any fish (fresh or smoked, canned as a third choice); sushi; tofu; tempeh; beans; avocado; organic eggs; free-range chicken; or free-range turkey. It's great to have any of these on a salad or with a salad. Be generous with a quality olive oil on your salad. Use bread, rice, or potatoes only when you must. Make them a side dish.

As with breakfast, lunch is not your time to calorie count. Just find your natural appetite and enjoy it.

Dinner is the meal where you have the greatest flexibility for macronutrient proportions. You don't need a meal dense in the slow-burning calories from fat or protein because the bulk of your energy needs have already been met for the day. Your calorie-burning metabolism is winding down. And for many people, a carbohydrate-centered meal in the evening can be relaxing, as opposed to stimulating. Listen to what your body is calling for. Even though this is the only meal to consider portion controlling, don't shortchange yourself on healthy fat. If you have a salad, use a gourmet olive oil. Oftentimes you'll end up eating more food or more carbohydrates than you need to if your body didn't get the fat it desired, and required, earlier in the day. If you're in the mood for a light dinner, or for no dinner, then follow the wisdom of your body. As with all meals, quality food is the key at dinner.

Exercise: Plan the Time and Size of Your Meals

Again, if weight loss and/or fatigue are the issues you'd like to address, or if you simply want to increase your energy level, try the following. Experiment with having a more substantial breakfast, make lunch your biggest meal whenever possible—or at least make it more robust if you usually eat lightly at this time. If you normally have a large dinner, try to make it smaller in size than it already is. Decrease it by approximately 10 to 20 percent. The goal is to eventually make dinner a smaller meal than your lunch.

If you find that you feel hungrier in the midmorning once you begin eating a larger breakfast, don't be upset with me. This is a great sign—it means your metabolism has increased. Your furnace is hotter and calling for more fuel, and you're recovering your natural appetite.

Timing is everything. Try to have your breakfast somewhere in the 6:30 to 9:00 AM range. Avoid having a later breakfast. Try to have your lunch in the 12:00 to 1:30 PM range. This is your peak metabolic time slot. Be aware that the later your breakfast, the more you'll be likely to push lunch past this time.

Do your best to eat dinner approximately four hours before bedtime. If you're the kind of person who eats very late and goes to bed right after meals, eating even an hour earlier will make a difference. Have a walk after a late dinner to enhance digestion. If you know you're going to have a late dinner, don't come to the table ravenous. Have a substantial snack about two hours before dinner. This will decrease your appetite and allow you to eat smaller portions.

Exercise: Plan Your Daily Meals and Snacks

Some people do fine on five to six smaller meals per day. Some just need three meals per day. Others get by on two. Some feel the need for snacks, while for many snacking isn't necessary.

We're all metabolically different. The only way to determine your unique needs relative to meal number is to experiment. If you have erratic meal patterns, switching to a solid schedule of three meals a day will be fabulous for you. If you don't have time for a more substantial relaxed lunch, it might be useful to have a smaller lunch and then a substantial late-afternoon snack. Think of it as two lunch meals. This is better for weight loss and energy level than skipping lunch and eating when you're ravenous and tired in the late afternoon. If you like, you can also experiment with having a midmorning and/or a midafternoon snack. Use the gut wisdom exercises from week 3 to feel what works best for you.

Tune in to your nutritional uniqueness. Try something different this week and note the results. If you want a light snack, use any fresh fruit or veggies. As best you can, cut down on pure carbohydrate snacks that are heavily processed and mass-produced—juices, sodas, candy, pretzels, chips, cookies, muffins, granola bars, and so on. Some great snack foods that are more substantial include organic nuts and seeds, trail mix, nut butter with fruit or veggies, organic yogurt, quality cheese with crackers or fruit, olives, bean dip, hummus, soup, and smoothies.

Exercise: Use Caffeine Wisely

Letting go of caffeine is a powerful way to reclaim your natural rhythm, which is the same as your healthiest and most robust metabolism. If you experience mood swings, energy dips, or have had problems with weight loss, this is your week for transforming your relationship to caffeine. This doesn't mean you should never have caffeine again or that caffeine is inherently bad. It's about you being the master of caffeine rather than it being the master of you. It's about finding your true energy. Either eliminate (best choice) or cut back to no more than one cup of coffee or other caffeinated beverage per day (next best choice). This includes caffeine-containing sodas, diet sodas, sports drinks, and black tea. (Even though decaf would be better in your experiment than regular, decaf still has caffeine in it.) If you must have coffee in the morning, have it with a meal. This will help modulate the insulin and blood-sugar spike—and subsequent drop—that occurs when you consume caffeine by itself.

Many of us are quite caffeine sensitive without even knowing it. That is, for most of us a little bit of caffeine goes a long way. For this reason I suggest you let go of all coffee for this week. If you feel you absolutely need a substitute, try green tea. It does contain caffeine and various chemicals related to caffeine, but it has less and yields a different effect on the nervous system. Green tea is also thermogenic—it enhances calorie burning but without raising your heart rate and blood pressure. Yerba mate is an herbal tea that's an excellent choice for a healthy and very lightly caffeinated drink that has a mildly invigorating effect. If desired, use a quality sweetener. You can also try herbal tea, or you can work on developing a taste for water.

Exercise: Get Regular Rest and Regular Play

This week see whether you can incorporate a regular relaxation period into the midafternoon of every day. Even fifteen minutes will be of good benefit. As best you can, close off the outside world, close your eyes, breathe, and recharge. This is not so much a sleep period as it is a time for meditative rest. (Be aware of the lighting in your home in the evening hours. Make it soft and soothing.) In many European and Latin American countries this period of rest is built into the lifestyle of the culture.

When we forget to allow time each day for regular rest and for regular play—and that means any activity that makes you smile—the food portion of our existence can take on a more weighty meaning. We put extra pressure on eating and expect it to give us something it ultimately cannot. Commit to experiencing some joy each day—playing with children, some form of fun exercise, dance, partner massage, chess, silly conversations, kisses. Whatever it is, it will benefit your biochemical well-being.

We've seen how nutrition and metabolism are intimately regulated by natural rhythms and how living a rhythmic life can rebalance us personally and emotionally. By bringing the power of rhythm into our relationship with food, the body finds its rightful place. Rhythm grounds the soul in the world.

Choosing rhythm means understanding that metabolism is not just about what you eat. It's about redesigning how you dance through your day. It's about balancing activity with rest, work with play, giving and receiving, thinking and feeling, head and heart. It's about choosing how you wish to live in the world.

❧ *Key Lessons*

- Alignment with the rhythms of life brings our metabolism into its fullest force.

- Digestive- and calorie-burning metabolism are strongest when the sun is highest in the sky (lunchtime) and weakest in the late evening hours.

- Skipping breakfast and lunch or under-eating at these meals can slow down metabolism and inhibit weight loss.

- Eating at irregular and unpredictable times each day may cause our digestive and calorie-burning metabolism to fall out of sync.

- Excessive consumption of refined carbohydrates causes a rhythmic meltdown, making the brain think it's summer and signaling the body to store fat.

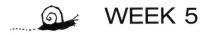 WEEK 5

The Metabolic Power of Pleasure

A firm defense of quiet material pleasure is the only way
to oppose the universal folly of Fast Life.

FROM THE SLOW FOODS INTERNATIONAL MANIFESTO

Vitamin P—pleasure—is a vital element that makes our meals nutritionally complete and makes life worth living. Like all organisms on the planet, we humans are genetically programmed to seek pleasure and avoid pain. A cat chasing a mouse is seeking pleasure; the unfortunate rodent is doing its best to avoid pain. Indeed, any behavior we can imagine can be seen as either of these or a mix of both. This is particularly apparent in light of our eating. When we eat, we are seeking the pleasure of food and avoiding the pain of hunger. Indeed, destiny has fashioned for us a body that's wired for joy.

The simple scientific equation for the profound biochemical effect of pleasure is this:

When you're turned on by food, you turn on metabolism.

In a study at the University of Texas, participants with very high cholesterol levels were placed on a low-fat diet; however, they were allowed to splurge every other day on a milkshake and a ham and cheese sandwich.[1] According to conventional wisdom they should have experienced a significant rise in blood cholesterol, but there was none. The only elevation they showed was that of enjoyment. Despite the high-fat content of the splurge foods, their cholesterol-raising effect was somehow mitigated by the chemistry of pleasure. It isn't hard to imagine that the splurges were the only relaxed and celebrated moments in an otherwise bland and stressful diet. And that decrease in fight-or-flight chemistry could have been, by itself, enough to lower cholesterol.

In another unusual study, researchers from Sweden and Thailand joined forces to determine how cultural preferences for food affects the absorption of iron from a meal.[2] A group of women from each country was fed a typical Thai meal—rice, veggies, coconut, fish sauce, and hot chili paste. As fate would have it, Thai women enjoy Thai food but Swedish women don't. This proved to be a crucial metabolic fact, because even though all the meals contained the exact same amount of iron, the Swedish women absorbed only half as much of the iron as the Thai women. To complete this phase of the study, both groups received a typical Swedish meal—hamburger, mashed potatoes, and string beans with the exact same iron content. Not surprisingly, the Thai women absorbed significantly less iron from the Swedish meal.

Next, the Thai women were separated into two groups. One group received the aforementioned Thai meal and the other was given the exact same meal as well—but that meal was first placed in a blender and turned to mush. Just imagine your favorite evening meal all whipped together into baby food. Even though the nutrient content of each meal was precisely equal, the women who ate the blender meal absorbed 70 percent less iron. Once again, the same results were seen for their Swedish counterparts who had their Swedish meal turned to a frappé.

The inescapable conclusion is that the nutritional value of a food is not merely given in the nutrients it contains but is dependent upon the synergistic factors that help us absorb those nutrients. Remove vitamin P, pleasure, and the nutritional value of our food plummets.

Add vitamin P and your meal is metabolically optimized. So if you're the kind of person who eats foods that are "good for you" even though you don't like them, or if you think you can have a lousy diet and make up for it by eating a strange-tasting vitamin-fortified protein bar, or if you've simply banished pleasure because you don't have enough time to cook or find a sumptuous meal—then you aren't doing yourself any nutritional favors. You're slamming shut the door on a key metabolic pathway.

In a fascinating animal study, scientists surgically destroyed the nerve centers of rats' brains that enable the rats to taste.[3] One group of rats was thus left with no ability to taste their food; a second group of normal, healthy, and luckier creatures who could still enjoy their meals was used as a control. Both groups were fed the exact same food, ate the same amounts, and were treated by researchers with the same manner of rat respect. In due time, every rat that couldn't taste died. The surprised scientists needed to find a cause of death so they autopsied the animals. They found that even though these rats ate the same healthy amount of food, they nevertheless died of clinical rat malnutrition. Their organs had wasted as if they'd been starved.

The moral of the story is that taste and pleasure are essential to life, more so perhaps than we could have ever imagined.

Chemical Clues to Pleasure

Consider the chemical cholecystokinin, CCK. This substance is produced by the body in response to protein or fat in a meal and performs a number of versatile functions. First, it directly aids digestion by stimulating the small intestines, pancreas, gallbladder, and stomach. Second, when it's released in the hypothalamus, part of the limbic area of the brain, it shuts down appetite. And last, CCK stimulates the sensation of pleasure in the cerebral cortex, the highest portion of the brain.

So in putting all this together we find that the same chemical that functions to metabolize our meal also tells us when it's time to finish that meal and makes us feel good about the entire experience. It shows us how pleasure, metabolism, and a naturally controlled appetite are interwoven to the core. Most people think that pleasure is completely separate from the nutritional process and serves no metabolic function. We believe that if a food makes us feel good the body is automatically stimulated to eat more. The actions produced by CCK in the brain tell us a whole new story.[4]

In the absence of pleasurable satiation, one of the chemicals that increases our appetite is neuropeptide Y. It tells us to search for food. It is naturally elevated in the morning, which makes sense because that's when the body is readying itself for action. Neuropeptide Y is also elevated whenever we are deprived of food. Its presence is particularly enhanced after dieting. Whenever we sink into a low blood sugar state—which usually means we are also in a low mood—neuropeptide Y is increased and stimulates us to consume carbohydrates.

So if you deny yourself the pleasure of food through low-calorie eating or if you restrict yourself to a fun-free diet, the body responds by chemically demanding pleasure and satisfaction. The lesson that neuropeptide Y teaches us is that we cannot escape the biological imperative to party and enjoy. No matter how stingy we are with eating, the body will not be denied.

The class of chemicals most people associate with pleasure are the endorphins. These substances are naturally produced throughout the body—most notably in the brain and the digestive system—and they exist, in part, to make us happy. The simple act of eating raises our levels of endorphins. This tells us that eating is an inherently pleasurable experience because biochemistry makes it so. What's most unusual about the endorphins is that not only are they molecules of pleasure, but they also stimulate fat mobilization. In other words, the same chemical that makes you feel good burns body fat. Furthermore, the greater the endorphin release in your digestive tract, the more blood and oxygen will be delivered there. This means increased digestion, assimilation, and ultimately greater efficiency in calorie burning.

Of course, I'm not telling you that you can eat a ton of dessert or junk food and that you'll burn it all as long as you feel pleasured. The point is that the chemistry of pleasure is intrinsically designed to fuel metabolism. When we make intelligent use of this biologic fact, our health can prosper. But if we don't receive the pleasure that body and soul call for each day and at every meal, we suffer. In the ancient and epic poem from India, the Mahabharata, we are told "Better to alight in flames, if only for a moment, than to smolder forever in unfulfilled desires."

Many of us claim to love food but when it's eaten too fast or without awareness or with a helping of guilt the central nervous system and the enteric nervous system both register only a minimum of pleasurable sensations. The result is that we are physiologically driven to eat more. We're compelled to hunt down the pleasure we never fully receive, even though it's continually within our grasp.

So if you're the kind of person who believes you can control your appetite and therefore lose weight by denying yourself pleasure, I suggest you reevaluate immediately. I have yet to meet one person who has successfully lost weight and kept it off by overcoming her or his natural, inborn drive to enjoy and celebrate food. Losing weight by limiting pleasure is like trying to stop smoking by not breathing. We can never increase the body's metabolic capacity by limiting what is essential to life.

Pleasure Catalyzes the Relaxation Response

The key to pleasure's powerful effect in balancing your appetite is that it promotes a physiologic relaxation response. The times we overeat most are when we're anxious, stressed, or unaware. A relaxed, pleasured eater has natural control. A stressed eater produces more circulating cortisol—the stress hormone we keep coming back to. What's amazing is that cortisol desensitizes us to pleasure. This is another of the brilliant functions of this chemical. When you're in a fight-or-flight response and trying to escape a hungry wolf, you don't want your brain to be in "feel good" mode and get sidetracked looking for chocolate. All of you needs to focus on survival.

So when cortisol desensitizes us to pleasure in our day-to-day stresses, we need to eat more food to feel the same amount of pleasure as when we're relaxed. This means that if you're afraid of pleasure or anxious about gaining weight or frightened to eat a dessert, you'll generate more cortisol. This chemical will swim through your bloodstream, numb you to pleasure, and ironically create the very self-fulfilling prophecy you feared from the beginning—"If I eat something fun, I won't be able to stop."

Can you see how our nutritional fears help create our metabolic reality?

Pleasure loves slow. It thrives in a warm, intimate, cozy space. It reveals its deepest secrets when we drop all pretensions of speed and allow timelessness and sensuality to breathe us back into each moment. The promise of speed—fast food, fast cars, fast service, fast results—has left us with a distinct blur of nothing. We then compensate with "hard"—we work hard, we play hard, we die hard—which altogether leaves us feeling exhausted and stiff. We might develop hardening of the arteries, a hardened heart, tight joints, or bones that crush under the weight of a high-impact life.

Pleasure is the essential antidote.

Putting Pleasure in Perspective

Epicurus is acknowledged as the ancient authority on the pleasures of the palate. We honor this Greek patriarch whenever we describe a dish as an "Epicurean delight." Few realize, though, that Epicurus was not some gluttonous pleasure junkie; he was actually a simple and austere man who chose his pleasures with great care, chose them wisely, and enjoyed them deeply. Perhaps his entire philosophy on pleasure is best summed up in his own words: "It is impossible to live pleasurably without living wisely, well, and, justly, and it is impossible to live wisely, well, and justly without living pleasurably."

I find that many people either fear the pleasure of food and do battle with it or constantly succumb to their food desires with little restraint.

Both do damage to body and psyche. Epicurus hints at a middle way. Using pleasure wisely means welcoming it with delight. It means including "healthy" pleasures and being moderate with the "unhealthy" ones so they do minimal damage at the least and leave us metabolically enhanced at the most. Unfortunately, many people get stuck in the notion that because many feel-good foods are "bad for you," eating them under any circumstances is detrimental. Such a view of nutrition is outdated.

Consider the case of chocolate. Some experts claim that chocolate is bad for you because it contains sugar and fat. Other experts will generously point out that chocolate contains magnesium and antioxidants, thereby making it good for you. Who's right?

Well, everyone. The answer to the question of who's right is in how much chocolate you eat. That is, the dose makes the poison. Small amounts of many substances or foods can be beneficial while larger amounts can be toxic. It's also about quality. Is your chocolate produced with integrity and made with fine ingredients? Do you eat your chocolate in a relaxed, aware, and celebrational manner? All these factors will contribute to determining the true nutritional value of your chocolate in a given moment. Yes, certain foods, such as fruits, are intrinsically healthy and can also provide us with pleasure. Yet many foods that would be considered "unhealthy" pleasures can be neutral to the body, and they can even be a metabolic "plus" when we consume them in a moderate dose and in a state of delight.

I'll speak more about the specifics of this shortly. First, consider this story.

Winnie, a thirty-four-year-old busy mother of three, came to see me with a food problem that had intensified ever since she had children—she constantly craved chocolate. No matter how much chocolate she had, she always wanted more and never felt satisfied. Winnie could happily discuss in detail all her favorite chocolate delicacies and why they excited her. She wanted to know how bad a problem this actually was—she wanted to rid herself of the problem but she still wanted to have chocolate in her life because she loved it so much.

Winnie was slender—she had never had a problem with weight,

and yet she was still concerned that if she gave in to her chocolate urge she would put on unwanted pounds. Furthermore, Winnie wondered if she mastered her craving and cut down on chocolate would she be able to indeed lose weight, even though she really didn't want to eat less chocolate or shed any pounds. Just wondering.

What surprised me about this wonderful lady was that when we started getting into the precise details of her daily chocolate rituals, I realized that she really didn't eat very much chocolate at all. Maybe a Milky Way after lunch, sometimes a single chocolate chip cookie after dinner. But most often she ate a no-fat, low-calorie chocolate pudding or frozen dessert after dinner. She never had chocolate more than twice a day; she usually ate it once a day, and some days she had none at all. Further discussion revealed that Winnie ate her chocolate fast. Oftentimes she felt stressed, and she never enjoyed food in general because she was in a constant rush to manage the schedules of three school-age kids. She was also chronically constipated, which I found significant but she had learned to live with.

I proposed to Winnie that perhaps she craved chocolate so much because she never really had any. Yes, she ate it, but she never fully received the pleasure she sought. She didn't generate a pleasure-chemistry release in her body and thus didn't fulfill her heart's desire or her cephalic phase digestive requirement. I explained that the higher her cortisol level—anxiety and stress—the lower her capacity to experience a physiologic pleasure response would be. Not only that, most of her chocolate was impotent. Many of her chocolate treats contained no fat. Research tells us that a 50/50 ratio of fat to sugar yields the greatest endorphin release in the body—"the real deal food orgasm."[5] The limp, fat-free chocolate pudding Winnie was eating couldn't truly perform and so was leaving her lust unsatisfied.

My prescription for Winnie was simple. Eat more chocolate. Eat real chocolate. Do the unthinkable and walk through the door of a gourmet chocolate shop and buy whatever you want. Plan a small dessert after every dinner or have a little chocolate after each lunch. Eat it slowly. Breathe. Indulge yourself with it.

Winnie followed this plan of action. In less than a month her chocolate "cravings" were gone and, pleasurably eating all the good chocolate she wanted, she didn't gain any weight. Chocolate was now a regular part of Winnie's diet that she loved and looked forward to but didn't obsess or worry about. Her relationship with pleasure had changed. She was now accepting it as part of her birthright rather than resisting it and holding herself back.

My favorite part of this story is that in the same time period Winnie's constipation cleared up and she went off laxatives for good. Some experts might tell you that it was the magnesium in the chocolate that gave her a laxative effect. Others would say that the extra fat could yield the same result. Skeptics would say it was just coincidence. But can you imagine how, at the very least, the chemistry of pleasure relaxed her chronically tense elimination system? Have no doubt. Opening to more pleasure can spark metabolism and return the body to its natural state of balance.

Health Is Pleasurable

What I'd like to suggest to you is that health, and by extension any action that promotes health, is inherently a deeply pleasurable experience. When you eat a food that's truly healthy for you, the body responds with a big biological "yes"—it activates a pleasure circuitry that is different from but no less potent than the pleasure pathways that are fired when you ingest a cheeseburger or french fries or an ice cream soda. A healthy food is one that your body recognizes as a biologic lock-and-key fit for promoting some aspect of full metabolic potential. A healthy food strikes a resonant chord deep within our cellular intelligence, the sound of which feels right and good.

Health is pleasurable. Healthy food is pleasurable. A food in its natural state is pleasurable. A food in its freshest state is pleasurable. A high-quality food is pleasurable. A creative dish is pleasurable. And any food that retains its personality, charm, and vital force is pleasurable.

Most of us don't have experiences like this all the time, and the reason is this: a fast-paced, fast-food, fast-exercise lifestyle closes a doorway of perception that decreases our pleasure threshold. We become acclimated to low-health, low-pleasure, mass-produced food. Our pleasure vocabulary decreases and we live, unaware, in a world in which our experience of joy never measures up to its true potential.

You might think you love nonfat frozen yogurt, or any diet food for that matter, but you really don't. It's not true love. You've settled for less; you've shortchanged your metabolism and fooled yourself into believing you're eating something of substance. Whenever someone tells me how much she loves a low calorie, no fat, artificially sweetened chocolate dessert, I say it's like sleeping with a guy you really don't want to be with but he's all that's around and the best you can do at the time so you'll settle for him. Eating fake pleasure foods is no different than sleeping with a stand-in lover. Yes, diet foods and junk foods can give great pleasure. But real foods give you even more.

Built for Sweet, Built for Fat

Another piece of the puzzle that joins pleasure with metabolic power is sweetness. Many people I meet believe they have a problem because they love sweets. Caught between this indestructible desire and its supposed result—weight gain—it's easy for us to feel unfairly duped by fate. The good news, though, is that if you have a sweet tooth and you think you have a problem because you have a sweet tooth, you don't. That's because we're built for sweet.

As you may recall from your earliest lessons in biology, humans have four types of taste buds on our tongues—sweet, salty, sour, and bitter. And bud for bud, we have more of the sweet variety of taste buds on our tongues than any of the others, and those vast amounts of sweet taste buds are mostly positioned toward the front and center portion of the tongue, where the greatest amount of our food tends to land.

And do you know what all those sweet taste buds are actually doing on your tongue? They are sitting there, waiting for something sweet.

That's the job of a sweet taste bud. It's vigilantly on the lookout for the opportunity to receive a sweet molecule and fire off an electro-chemical signal to the brain for the sole purpose of turning you on. And indeed, your sweet taste buds *must* do this. Imagine what would happen if you were blindfolded for a day and denied the sense of sight. It may be a novel experience for the first few minutes, but it likely soon becomes unpleasant and perhaps even unbearable. The senses of the body—sight, sound, touch, taste, smell—must be fulfilled. If we "blind-folded" our sweet taste buds by not giving ourselves the pleasure of a sweet food, or if we continually use artificial sweeteners, disharmony is the result, and we'll crave sweetness even more.

Incidentally, the same concept holds true for salt. Do you think God gave you highly complex taste buds for salt just to torture you and raise your blood pressure?

The point is not to consume toxic amounts of sugar and salt. Any-thing that is pleasurable in small amounts becomes painful in large doses. Your favorite song played over and over for hours would be irri-tating. Hanging around your best friend for two weeks straight might ruin the friendship. We must monitor our dosage of pleasure as we would any other powerful drug. But you must also make sure you're get-ting enough.

From an evolutionary perspective, then, sweetness is a biological reward. It gives us a reason to keep living. Have you ever noticed that after eating a meal you just want a little something sweet, and that it can even be a small taste of someone's dessert that could satisfy you? That's your central nervous system calling for vitamin P—pleasure—through it's specialized nerve endings called sweet taste buds that often need just a minimum of excitation to satisfy this key component of the cephalic phase digestive requirement.

Another obstacle that prevents us from receiving the full metabolic power of pleasure is how we do fat. Specifically, our erroneous concepts about the biology of fat has many of us fearing the fat in food, follow-ing a low-fat diet, and suffering consequences with health that we couldn't have imagined. Deny yourself the pleasure of fat and you deny the full power of metabolism.

We've seen that healthy fats are essential to life. As is often the case in nature, when something is required for our biological existence, it feels good. Take a drink of some cool water when you're dehydrated and you'll feel the reward. Take a deep breath after you've been submerged too long and you'll experience immediate delight. Eat a fat-containing food and you'll feel satisfied and fulfilled. That's because fat is required by the body, and fulfilling requirements feels good. Pleasure sensations are genetically programmed to occur on the tongue, throughout the gut, and in the brain. Fat, pleasure, and survival are therefore inseparable. They make up a holy trinity of the body. But if you're like most Americans, you're probably pulling this trinity apart on a daily basis and suffering the consequences.

Even though the body needs fat for survival, if you think it's bad, you'll avoid it as best you can. But since fat is inherently pleasurable it will call to you again and again like a distant voice in your nutritional wilderness, tempting you to break a rule that you think is cosmic law but has been erroneously created by highly fallible nutritionists, doctors, and experts. If you're successful in eating an extremely low-fat diet, you'll eventually develop signs of clinical or subclinical fat deficiency. Some of the signs of this condition include weakness, irritability, fatigue, dry or oily skin, acne, funky hair, dandruff, psoriasis, brittle nails, digestive complaints, depression, moodiness, redness around the eyes, susceptibility to colds, joint pains, constipation, and (bizarrely enough) weight gain or an inability to lose weight.

In a study at Bowman-Gray University, scientists separated monkeys into two groups. The first group received a regular-fat monkey diet while the second group received a no-fat monkey diet. After a period of time, the researchers observed that the monkeys eating the normal amount of fat behaved like normal monkeys—playful and active. The monkeys on the no-fat diet became agitated and violent, with some monkeys nearly killing each other.

If you know someone following a no-fat diet, I suspect this information might be very useful, at least for your own protection. And incidentally, none of the monkeys on the no-fat diet lost any weight.

Pleasure Heals

Louise, a fifty-one-year-old legal secretary, made an appointment to see me because she was bored with her diet and wanted some new ideas and menu suggestions. She described herself as the kind of person who eats the same thing all the time.

Louise's diet was as follows. Breakfast consisted of coffee and half of a bagel with margarine. Lunch was a salad with nonfat dressing and nonfat cottage cheese with a diet soda. In the late afternoon she had a nonfat frozen yogurt—this was her favorite food moment of the day. Dinner was either skinless chicken with vegetables and rice or a Lean Cuisine frozen meal. Dessert was nonfat cookies. No wonder she was bored.

But boredom was the least of Louise's problems. She admitted she'd been following this eating plan for almost two years to lose weight and only a few pounds came off. Even though she wasn't seeking any advice from me about health, she shared that since following this diet her hair had become brittle, her skin was extremely dry, she was fatigued, she had frequent colds, and she was constantly hungry. Louise's diet was virtually fat free and she was paying the price!

Even though I explained in precise detail how all her symptoms pointed to clinical fat deficiency, Louise was nevertheless appalled at my recommendation that she put fresh peanut butter on her bagel and olive oil in her salad, that she eat wild salmon instead of Lean Cuisine, and choose real ice cream over the nonfat counterfeit kind. Louise insisted that she enjoyed nonfat foods and couldn't possibly eat anything "fatty" because she wouldn't be able to stop and would gain weight.

Louise's biggest fear wasn't of fat. She was most afraid of pleasure. Her relationship with food was a mirror of her relationship with life. She wasn't just bored with eating, she was bored with living. Louise spoke of how she was in a rut with her job, her marriage, and her social life. She had little joy in her life, and in the same way that she had convinced herself that her job was at least worth staying at, she had cajoled herself into believing that fat-free foods tasted good. The less fat she ate the less pleasure she felt and the more her body developed symptoms of pain and dysfunction. So the biggest challenge we faced together wasn't to convince Louise to eat fat—which was certainly difficult enough—but to cultivate trust in pleasure.

Working together, Louise and I devised a plan to slowly reintroduce healthy fat into her diet. As she saw some of her symptoms dissipate, and as she realized she could eat a peanut or an olive and not gain weight, Louise grew more confident with this approach. Over the course of a year she transformed into a happier, positive, and vibrant woman. All of her fat-deficiency symptoms cleared. Her skin was healthy, her hair was shiny, and her energy returned. She admitted that for the first time since she was a child, eating was fun.

Most intelligent clinicians would say that the addition of essential fatty acids to Louise's diet was directly responsible for alleviating her symptoms. To this I would agree 100 percent, but I would add this important fiat: Pleasure heals. It isn't the mere chemistry of fat metabolism that made Louise's appearance bright and shiny. The acceptance and expression of pleasure also helped to bring out her true radiance.

Can you see the fascinating connection between nutritional metabolism, pleasure, and beauty? Do you understand how these are mind-body-spirit phenomena? Can you think of areas in your own life where opening the door to pleasure might yield a similar breakthrough?

When pleasure is made forbidden we never truly receive it. The body yearns for it and we do great battle against it or we give it ineffective substitutes—low-fat, low-taste, mass-produced foods that leave us unfulfilled. It's time for a new approach.

Week 5: Your Primary Task

This week is your opportunity to deepen into the pleasures of eating. It's a time when you can focus on the joyous sensations of food, of dining, and of the warm and welcome feelings that wash over the body after eating a meal that is supportive of your health. Deepening to pleasure is about getting out of your head and into the sensuality of every cell. It's your chance to explore and experiment with the wise use of bliss.

Exercise: Healthy Food Pleasure Inventory

Your week begins with the most trustworthy pleasures—the healthy ones. In your journal, write an inventory of all the foods that you've learned (or that you firmly believe or strongly intuit) are healthy for you *and* have the added bonus of delivering to you a pleasurable experience. This list might include fruit, fish, nuts, a macrobiotic meal, a fresh juice, an omelet, a smoothie, a favorite salad, chicken soup, a bowl of oatmeal, fresh coconut, a cup of tea, a glass of wine, garlic—anything. Keep in mind that you are accessing both your acquired intellectual knowledge and your own bodily experience, so let go of trying to know with absolute universal certainty whether a food is truly healthy or not.

Your task this week is simply to include each day at least three of these foods or ingredients in your day's meals.

Eat with awareness, focusing on the pleasurable sensations on your tongue, in your belly, and wherever else pleasure registers in your body. Notice the unique ways that a healthy pleasure occurs to you. Does it leave you feeling lighter? More satisfied? Happy with yourself? Does it give you a sense of accomplishment? Can you intuit the long-term benefits it can confer on your health?

As you allow the pleasure of wholesome, quality, conscientiously prepared foods to reveal itself more fully, you'll find that your tolerance for low-quality food decreases. You'll have cultivated a higher taste that's in greater alignment with your metabolic needs. The end result is that you'll have more pleasurable foods to choose from because the size of your food harem will have multiplied, and you'll make better overall choices about the foods you pick to nourish and entertain yourself.

This next exercise is about learning how to make the "unhealthy" pleasures work for you. It's for extra credit, so do it only if you're interested in trusting and believing in yourself.

Exercise: Forbidden Food Pleasure Inventory

Take a few moments to write down in your journal everything in the food universe that turns you on, no matter how forbidden or how unhealthy you or anyone else believes these foods to be. Include in your list specific foods that give great pleasure, specific meals, specific brands, and any other details that are important to painting the full pleasure picture.

Once your list is complete, study it. Observe your reactions to what you've written. What does this list teach you about you? How often do you eat these foods? When do you tend to eat them? With whom? Which ones elicit in you the most desire? Which ones cause you the greatest guilt?

Your extra-credit assignment for this week is to eat one or two of these forbidden foods or meals. Rather than put these pleasures in the nutritional doghouse, put them on a pedestal instead—worship them by bringing them down to Earth and onto the table for a special occasion. Eat slowly, taking your time and releasing all guilt. Celebrate.

After you enjoy your forbidden pleasure, notice how you feel. Does your body react to this food in any way? Does the food enhance your energy level or drain you of energy? What happens to your mood? How do you feel the next morning? Check in with your gut wisdom. Should this food be excluded from your diet or is it really something you need? Can you eat it occasionally and make it work? The choice is yours.

If you know you're the kind of person who needs a forbidden pleasure each day, then make plans to have your one treat at a specific time each day, for example after lunch or dinner or in the late afternoon. Agreeing that your reward is forthcoming at a regular time will take the edge off any worries about not getting what you want and will give you something to look forward to. If it's a poor-quality high-fat and high-sugar delight that you absolutely can't give up, have it once or twice a month. If that's not truly enough, bump it up to an amount you can live with.

As best you can, replace your forbidden pleasure foods with higher quality and organic versions. Decide on a portion size that will make you feel that you've gotten the pleasure you want yet leaves you feeling good, as though you respected your natural limits. Remember, there are no formulas for amounts that fit for every person. This is about empowering yourself in your relationship with food and pleasure. The result will be an empowered metabolism. If your nutritionist or health expert thinks this is unsound advice, give that person a hug and send some chocolates.

Choose Pleasure

No matter what you eat, your ultimate goal for week 5 is to make 85 to 100 percent of your meals and snacks pleasurable. Everything that passes your lips will be an opportunity for sensual delight. The strategy to help you get there is to ask yourself this one simple question as you eat: "Is this pleasurable?"

If the answer is yes, then enjoy. If the answer is no, then take a moment to consider your options. You can either change what you eat or you can change you, the eater. Changing yourself first can elicit more pleasure from the food. This means eating with increased awareness and in a relaxed manner and momentarily letting go of all concerns so you can be present with your meal. Taste whatever you eat as deeply as you can to find the healing pleasures hidden within it. Choose to experience the joy of eating every time you eat.

If a food delivers little pleasure even when fully savored, then you may be making a nutritionally unwise choice or the quality of the chosen food may be too low. Attending to the food we eat and sensing it with relaxed discrimination often reveals that we don't truly enjoy many of the foods we choose. Check in with your gut wisdom, your enteric nervous system, to discover more insights about these foods and whether or not you should eliminate them.

We know that certain foods that fail to deliver pleasure in the moment will likely yield health benefits later in the day (or later in life). For many people, and especially children, this pertains especially to vegetables, salads, whole grains, homemade soups, seaweeds, and medicinal herbs and teas. Again, check in with your enteric nervous system to see where a particular food stands. Oftentimes, knowing that a food will yield a health benefit is a pleasure in itself.

Likewise, many foods that yield pleasure in the short term can detract from our pleasure later in the day (or in life). Excess sugar, coffee, and fried foods are typical examples. And yet, eaten occasionally and in moderate quantities, such foods may be neutral or even beneficial. Once again, the wisdom of your enteric nervous system is the final word when faced with such choices.

The secret to activating the metabolic power of pleasure in your body is trust. Just as you learn over time to trust a friend or a business partner, pleasure needs to be trusted as well. Drop your suspicions and allow body and soul what they require. Trust in pleasure, trust in your ability to experience it and be able to control yourself, and trust that even if you overeat a pleasurable food and feel guilty or sick, you can still recover, set yourself straight, and continuously rediscover a place of joyful harmony with food. Give pleasure the trust it deserves and the rewards will be forthcoming.

Exercise: Personal Pleasure Inventory

Next, write a list that includes everything else in existence that brings you pleasure—people, places, vacations, topics of conversation, a favorite chair, a perfect evening, a beauty product, a bath, a favorite magazine, anything legal or illegal, sensual delights, sexual delights, flowers, silly things, simple things. If you've never taken a total inventory of that which delights you, be thorough and daring. Notice how some pleasures on your list are easily claimed and acknowledged by you while others may seem taboo.

Once you've bared your soul and told all your earthly pleasures on paper, read through that list as if you were a social scientist studying yourself. Become more interested in the topic of you and pleasure. Does this list teach you anything that you didn't know about yourself? Which are the pleasures you most steadfastly allow yourself? Which are the ones that seem more absent from your life? Which are the greatest? The simplest? The ones you long for the most? Which are the ones that come most natural to you? Which are more "problematic"?

Oftentimes, receiving pleasure from food takes on unfair importance when we're shortchanging ourselves in regard to pleasure in other areas of life. By spreading around the love, we take the pressure off of our meals to perform. This week, in addition to eating one or two "forbidden" foods, include a nonfood pleasure in your life at least twice each day. Allow yourself to feel enriched by that which predictably brings you delight. In addition, choose a pleasure that you can enjoy once this week, the kind whose effects can linger for days. This could be a massage, a visit with a special friend, a long-distance phone call, or an outing to an inspirational spot.

Pleasure is, perhaps, the ultimate reward. Biologically, it grants us greater probability for survival, enhanced health, and a vitalized metabolism. Psychologically, its bounty is a sense of well-being, connectedness, and plain old fun. Spiritually, pleasure's reward is the discovery of the sacred essence hidden within all of earthly creation. No other nutrient can restore the radiance to body, heart, and soul as this one does. It's time to welcome pleasure back to the table.

Key Lessons

- A pleasurable experience of a meal enhances nutrient absorption.

- A nonpleasurable experience decreases it.

- Pleasure catalyzes the relaxation response, promoting parasympathetic dominance and full digestive force.

- Excess cortisol production from stress or anxiety desensitizes us to pleasure. This causes us to eat more food during times of stress to register the food's pleasurable effects.

- We are genetically programmed to desire and enjoy the sweet taste and to desire and enjoy fat. Eating quality versions of these promotes a healthier metabolism.

- The way we experience pleasure with food is a mirror of how we experience pleasure in life.

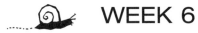 WEEK 6

The Metabolic Power of Thought

Thoughts rule the world.

RALPH WALDO EMERSON

One of the most fundamental building blocks of nutritional metabolism is neither vitamin, mineral, nor molecule. It's our relationship with food. It's the sum total of our innermost thoughts and feelings about what we eat. Consider the word *relationship*. Each of us, whether we know it or not, is in an intimate, lifelong, committed union with eating. It's not by accident that the same words that describe our relationships with people equally characterize our relationships with food—love, hate, pleasure, pain, expectations, disappointments, excitement, boredom, uncertainty, change. This relationship with food is as deep and revealing as any we might ever have.

The great Sufi poet Rumi once remarked "The satiated man and the hungry man do not see the same thing when they look upon a loaf of bread." And Al Capone, noted gangster, astutely observed, "When I sell liquor, it's called bootlegging; when my patrons serve it on silver trays on Lake Shore Drive, it's called hospitality." Indeed, how each of us thinks about eating is so profoundly relative that if a group of us were looking at the same plate of food, no two people would see the same thing.

Say, for example, we were examining a plate of pasta, chicken, and salad. A woman wanting to lose weight would see calories and fat. She'd respond favorably to the salad or chicken but would view the pasta with fear. An athlete trying to gain muscle mass would look at the same meal and see protein. She'd focus on the chicken and look past the other foods. A pure vegetarian would see the distasteful sight of a dead animal and wouldn't touch anything on the plate. A chicken farmer, on the other hand, would be proud to see a good piece of meat. Someone trying to heal a disease through diet would see either potential medicine or potential poison, depending upon whether or not the plate of food is permissible on her chosen diet. A scientist studying nutrient content in food would see a collection of chemicals.

What's amazing is that each of these eaters will metabolize this same meal quite differently in response to her unique thoughts. In other words, what you think and feel about a food is as important a determinant of its nutritional value and its effect on body weight as the actual nutrients themselves.

Does this sound unbelievable? Here's how the science works.

How Your Brain Eats

The information highway of brain, spinal cord, and nerves is like a telephone system through which your mind communicates with your digestive organs. Let's say you're about to eat an ice cream cone. The notion and image of that ice cream occurs in the higher center of the brain—the cerebral cortex. From there, information is relayed electrochemically to the limbic system, which is considered the "lower" portion of the brain. The limbic system regulates emotions and key physiological functions such as hunger, thirst, temperature, sex drive, heart rate, and blood pressure. Within the limbic system is a pea-sized collection of tissues known as the hypothalamus, which integrates the activities of the mind with the biology of the body. In other words, it takes sensory, emotional, and thought input and transduces this information into physiological responses.[1] This is nothing short of a miracle.

If the ice cream is your favorite flavor—say, chocolate—and you consume it with a full measure of delight, the hypothalamus will modulate this positive input by sending activation signals via parasympathetic nerve fibers to the salivary glands, esophagus, stomach, intestines, pancreas, liver, and gallbladder. Digestion will be stimulated and you'll have a fuller metabolic breakdown of the ice cream while burning its calories more efficiently.

If you're feeling guilty about eating the ice cream or judging yourself for eating it, the hypothalamus will take this negative input and send signals down the sympathetic fibers of the autonomic nervous system. This initiates inhibitory responses in the digestive organs, which means you'll be eating your ice cream but not fully metabolizing it. It may stay in your digestive system longer, which can diminish your population of healthy gut bacteria and increase the release of toxic by-products into the bloodstream. Furthermore, inhibitory signals in the nervous system can decrease your calorie-burning efficiency, which would cause you to store more of your guilt-infused ice cream as body fat. So the thoughts you think about the food you eat instantly become reality in your body via the central nervous system.

Our thoughts also directly impact some of the most powerful metabolic chemicals we know of—hormones. As information about the ice cream travels from the cerebral cortex to the hypothalamus, it exerts its influence upon the pituitary, the master gland of the endocrine system that sits at the base of the brain. The pituitary gland transmits information from the realm of the mind into the language of hormones. It relays hormonal signals to the pancreas, adrenals, parathyroid gland, kidneys, and thyroid gland. Remember the cephalic phase insulin response that can cause you to gain weight just by thinking about ice cream? That's the endocrine pathway operating via the pancreas.

Or consider the importance of the thyroid gland. Many people already know that a well-functioning thyroid is a key requirement for a healthy metabolism. If you're not producing enough thyroid hormone you'll likely feel tired, sluggish, or depressed. And you'd probably feel that no matter how little food you eat you still won't lose weight.

Interestingly enough, a healthy attitude toward the ice cream promotes thyroid hormone release, which increases your output of digestive hormones and the motility of the digestive tract and revs up the metabolic rate of almost every cell in the body. All this not by taking a thyroid pill but by loving and respecting your ice cream cone!

On the other hand, anxious thoughts about the ice cream would inhibit thyroid hormone, which translates to decreased metabolism and increased fat deposition. It can also trigger stress-hormone release, which as we've seen means inefficient digestion, nutrient wasting, calcium loss, and weight gain.

So we've now seen that not only does eating under stress diminish metabolism but thinking stressful thoughts has the same results. The brain doesn't distinguish between a real stressor or an imagined one. If you sat in a room all by yourself, happy and content, and started thinking about the guy who did you wrong five years ago, if that story still carries a charge for you your body would quickly adapt to the physiologic stress-state—increased heart rate and blood pressure, decreased digestive function.

Any guilt about food, shame about the body, or judgment about health are considered stressors by the brain and are immediately transduced into their electrochemical equivalents in the body. You could eat the healthiest meal on the planet, but if you're thinking toxic thoughts the digestion of your food goes down and your fat storage metabolism goes up. Likewise, you could be eating a nutritionally challenged meal, but if your head and heart are in the right place, the nutritive power of your food will be increased.

Placebo on a Plate

To fully appreciate the power of mind over metabolism, let's take a fresh look at one of the most compelling phenomena in science: the placebo effect. Here's my favorite example of this extraordinary force.

In 1983, medical researchers were testing a new chemotherapy treatment.[2] One group of cancer patients received the actual drug being tested while another group received a placebo—a fake, harmless, inert chemical substance. As you may know, pharmaceutical companies are required by law to test all new drugs against a placebo to determine the true effectiveness, if any, of the product in question. In the course of this study, no one thought twice when 74 percent of the cancer patients receiving the real chemotherapy exhibited one of the more common side effects of this treatment: they lost their hair. Yet, quite remarkably, 31 percent of the patients on the placebo chemotherapy—an inert saltwater injection—also had an interesting side effect: they lost their hair, too. Such is the power of expectation. The only reason that those placebo patients lost their hair is because they believed they would. Like many people, they associated chemotherapy with going bald.

So if the power of the mind is strong enough to make our hair fall out when taking a placebo, what do you think happens when we think to ourselves "This cake is fattening, I really shouldn't be eating it," or "I'm going to eat this fried chicken but I know it's bad for me," or "I enjoy eating my salad because it's really healthy"?

Certainly I'm not saying we can eat poison without any harm if we believe it's good for us. I'm suggesting that what we believe about any substance we consume can powerfully influence how it affects the body. Every day, millions of people eat and drink while thinking strong and convincing thoughts about their meal. Consider some of the foods you've given strong associations to:

"Salt will raise my blood pressure."
"Fat will make me fatter."
"Sugar will rot my teeth."
"I can't make it through the day without my cup of coffee."
"This meat will raise my cholesterol level."
"This calcium will build my bones."

To a certain degree, some of these statements may be true. But is it possible that we are instigating these effects? And if these effects *are* the inherent result of eating these foods, can you see how we can enhance those results with the potency of our expectations?

The placebo effect is not some rare and unusual creature. Its appearance is quite commonplace. Researchers have estimated that 35 to 45 percent of all prescription drugs may owe their effectiveness to placebo power and that 67 percent of all over-the-counter medications, such as headache remedies, cough medicines, and appetite suppressants, are also placebo based. In some studies the response to placebos is as high as 90 percent.[3]

It amazes me that no one in the scientific community has made the obvious connection between placebo power and food. Indeed, the placebo effect is built into the nutritional process. It is profoundly present on a day-to-day basis every time we eat. Simply put, the placebo force is how your metabolism responds to thoughts, feelings, and expectations. It's like phoning in a prescription to your own inner nutritional pharmacy. What we believe is alchemically translated into the body through nerve pathways, the endocrine system, neuropeptide circulation, the immune network, and the digestive tract.

In one fascinating study researchers found that subjects who were given a placebo and were told it was vitamin C had significantly fewer colds than subjects who were given real vitamin C and told it was a placebo.[4] In a Cornell University study of an appetite-suppressing drug, patients who were given this drug but were told nothing about its side effects showed no change in calorie intake or body weight. When they were told the drug would suppress their appetites they began to eat less and shed pounds. In fact, numerous studies have shown that placebos are as effective in reducing appetite as any over-the-counter drug.[5]

Recall the discussion in week 1 about the metabolic power of relaxation and the French. Many people who've visited such countries as Portugal, Spain, Holland, France, Denmark, Sweden, and Brazil have noticed that many women in these nations show little interest in eating nonfat foods, counting calories, or restricting their pastry intake. Furthermore, they don't relate to treadmills and jogging and they eat more fat than American women, and yet they're happier, healthier, and thinner. They believe the foods they eat will have a positive effect on their bodies. Compare this with the many American women who are culturally conditioned to worry about grams of fat, who fear food and ceaselessly diet. Can you see how such thoughts become a self-fulfilling metabolic prophecy through the power of the placebo?

Good Food, Bad Food

There's one particular nutritional thought I'd like to alert you to that lingers in the minds of many, is the most metabolically damaging, and is best removed from our mental diet. The outdated thought is this: Some foods are good, some foods are bad.

Strangely enough, the notion of good foods and bad ones is largely unscientific. As we've seen, the metabolic value of any foodstuff is profoundly influenced by factors that aren't inherent in the food but issue forth from the eater—relaxation, quality, awareness, pleasure, and so on.

In truth, though, there's no such thing as a good or bad food.

Allow me to explain.

Yes, it's clear that certain foods will enhance your health while others will detract from it. When I say to you there's no such thing as a good food or bad food, I'm pointing out that no food is *morally* good or bad. In other words, no one can say they've uncovered an evil conspiracy between bacon and eggs to raise our cholesterol. Nor has anyone come forward claiming to have seen heavenly angels flying about their salad. Food is morally neutral. So is every other object in the universe. Is a baseball bat good or bad? It depends on how you use it. It can be used to can hit a home run and thus make thousands of fans deliriously happy or it can be a tool of destruction, used to smash someone's car window and ruin her day.

Is a food good or bad? It depends on how you use it. This distinction is of the utmost importance if you wish to have even the slightest chance of a happy relationship with food and with your body. So much of the misery that pollutes our emotional atmosphere around eating comes from the consequences of moralizing about food. That's because if you choose to label a food "bad," what does that imply about you if you eat it? It implies that you're a bad person. And as everyone knows, bad people need to be punished, and severely, so they don't want to do bad things ever again. When we moralize about food in this way we put ourselves in the unusual position of being both the guilty party and the judge. We might sentence ourselves to a miserable low-calorie diet, to extra helpings of punishing exercise, or maybe just to some good old-fashioned guilt, shame, and self-abuse. All of which, of course, creates a physiologic stress-state, and you know what that means for metabolism. My point is that the various remedies we concoct for our crimes actually create a far worse result than the crime itself. (Politicians and law-makers please take note.)

Something else happens when we label a food good or bad. We stop the process of questioning and discovery. We stop being curious. If you were told by a colleague that the new guy in your office is a jerk, you'd have him labeled. You might never get to know him and so you might lose out on a potential best friend. The same goes with food. If we label sugar as bad, we stop asking detailed questions to learn about sugar's nuances and complexities. Are all kinds of sugar undesirable or are some kinds better than others? Can eating sugar with other foods mitigate any of sugar's negative effects? Does sugar react differently in children's bodies than in adults'? Moralizing about anything or anyone severely limits our knowledge of the world and causes us to dwell in fear, ignorance, and judgment.

This situation is best exemplified with alcohol. Americans have a peculiar moral relationship with this substance. We drink it, we enjoy it, we abuse it in staggering proportions, and our scientists can't decide if it's a medicine or a poison. (Hint: It's both.)

So is wine good or bad? It depends on how you use it. Only you can know the right dose for you. Some people feel fine with a few glasses in the evening. Others remark that they used to tolerate alcohol quite well but now a little bit makes them tired. These are some of the natural changes the body undergoes that only you and I can account for. You are the expert on you. And as you allow yourself to develop this natural expertise, along with your curiosity, you'll become more expert at knowing when to use and trust the expert advice of others.

When we talk about the power of mind over food we are entering new scientific territory. Researchers for the most part have been silent on this topic because there's little interest in it and it's a difficult area in which to design a reliable study. For me, though, the proof comes from the front lines. Working with individuals and watching their health change or their weight transform simply by shifting their negative beliefs is the real living proof.

Krista, a thirty-seven-year-old administrative assistant, was a lifelong yo-yo dieter whose weight fluctuated between 140 and 152 pounds. When dieting, Krista ate what she considered the "good foods"—a yogurt at breakfast, a salad at lunch, a piece of chicken at dinner, and no sweets or desserts. At such times she felt in control and happy with herself. But if she dared to stray off her diet and yield to the "bad foods"—bread, ice cream, pizza, and junk-food snacks—she'd lose control, punish herself, live in anxiety, and secretly binge. She'd gain weight and lose her dignity. In Krista's mind she was either a good girl or a bad girl, each entirely in relationship to her diet. There was no middle ground. Krista desperately wanted to stop dieting and stay at her desired weight, but after almost two decades without lasting success, she felt hopeless.

I suggested to Krista that her best chance to have what she wanted would be to focus on what needed to change most—her thinking. Specifically, she needed to discard one set of thoughts: the "good food/bad food" business. This was the root of her problem, and it led to a battle with biology that caused a cascade of harmful behaviors that resulted in increasing body fat, not decreasing it.

I asked Krista to act as if foods were neither good nor bad but were morally neutral. I asked her to stop seeing herself as bad if she ate a bad food. This meant no more self-punishment. I also asked her to take on a new thought about food—that it was her friend. Discarding old thoughts and trying on new ones is like changing clothes. It's no big deal—you just need to try it. Krista agreed to do her best to welcome food and relate with it in a new way. In doing so, she also opened the door to work with and receive the metabolic benefits of relaxation, awareness, pleasure, rhythm, and quality. Krista eventually succeeded because she released a way of thinking that had her locked in a deeply held physiologic stress, the same kind of stress that raises cortisol and insulin and deposits weight.

Her weight finally stabilized in the low 140s. Most importantly, Krista felt empowered and free to enjoy food and had regained her self-respect. And it all began by changing a single, metabolically limiting thought.

Motivation, Exercise, and Metabolism

Here is one more story I'd like to share about the metabolic power of thought. It's about two clients who provided me with one of the big "aha's" of my professional career. Early on in my nutritionist practice, a forty-eight-year-old female lawyer named Toni was referred to me by a local physician in New York City. He warned me that she was a difficult patient who was trying to lose weight but couldn't. The doctor did numerous tests but found nothing wrong with Toni; he had suggested various diets and she hadn't lost a single pound. The highlight of this case was that Toni was a marathon runner. She ate a paltry 1,300 calories per day, she ran eight to ten miles a day during the work week and about fifteen miles on Saturday, and she was a legitimate candidate for losing fifteen pounds.

When Toni walked into my office I was surprised to see that she looked absolutely nothing like a marathon runner. She was short, plump, and high-strung. I'd never seen someone in such a panic about her weight. Toni had spent thousands of dollars on blood tests and to have her body poked and probed to find something wrong but was given a clean bill of health. This highly intelligent, super-successful woman was absolutely beside herself that she could be exercising so much, eating so little, and seeing no results after a year of training.

With the right questions I quickly determined that, contrary to my suspicions, Toni was telling the truth. She was really running and she was really starving herself.

I was quite confident I could help. Toni's diet was clearly deficient in protein, fat, and calories, which was putting her in a survival response and slowing down her metabolism. She ate fast, received no pleasure from food, and seldom had a nourishing meal. We had lots to work on. I told Toni it would take eight sessions over a two-month period to begin to shift her weight. I explained that she had to eat more food, including more fat and protein, and she needed to learn to relax and receive pleasure from food.

Toni looked at me as though I was insane and insisted that if she ate anything more than she was eating now she would most certainly gain weight. She admitted that she didn't believe me but acknowledged that she was at the end of her rope and would try anything. And she made me promise that she wouldn't gain a pound on her new regime. Without my asking, she wrote a check for all eight sessions and walked out of the office more agitated than when she walked in.

At the end of two weeks Toni weighed six pounds more and threatened to sue me. Her worst nightmare had come true. I was devastated. Her lawyer was sending me intimidating letters. I quickly returned Toni's money, apologized every way possible, and the whole affair blew over. But I never forgot her and remained mystified about her case.

Fast forward to seven years later. A woman comes into my office who could be the sister of this marathon runner that I've never forgotten. Sheila was yet another high-achieving woman, a stockbroker in her late forties—short, plump, healthy, a low-calorie and high-mileage marathoner who couldn't lose a pound. I would have instantly referred her to someone else but a number of her close friends who had come to see me had all shared their wonderful success stories, so Sheila was eager to work with me. I couldn't send her away, nor could I think of any strategies other than the unsuccessful ones I tried seven years ago. It seemed as though the universe was entertaining itself by having a good laugh at my expense.

I gave Sheila the same advice I had given Toni: eat more food, especially more fat and protein, and slow down when eating. In two weeks Sheila gained four pounds. I felt like a criminal and was ready to surrender myself to the authorities. Surprisingly though, she wasn't upset or deterred. She was so inspired and positive about how her friends had benefited from working with me that she felt certain I could figure this out.

This is where the "aha" came in. An exercise physiologist friend explained to me that intense exercise can closely mimic the stress response. Yes, aerobic exercise is great for us and has a long list of wonderful metabolic benefits. I know this because I personally place a high value on working out. But in the wrong context exercise can wear us down, elevating cortisol and insulin levels, generating inflammatory chemicals, and locking us into a survival metabolism in which we vigorously store fat and arrest the building of muscle. According to conventional wisdom, weight is a function of calories in and calories out. So the more you exercise the more weight you will supposedly lose. But in reality, the exercise story is never so black-and-white. Kenneth Cooper, M.D., the granddaddy of the fitness movement in America and a previous proponent of intense workouts, has done a complete about-face concerning vigorous aerobic exercise. His research findings at the Cooper Aerobics Center in Dallas, Texas, were so astounding that I think anyone who does high-intensity workouts should take note. Basically, Kenneth Cooper discovered that low- to moderate-intensity exercise for only thirty minutes three or four times per week was the best prescription for health, weight maintenance, and fitness.[6]

On our next visit I asked Sheila why she ran marathons. She said she needed to do something for fitness and she liked running. I asked her if she really wanted to run so much or if there were other forms of fitness she would prefer. She was uncomfortable with my questioning and was taken aback when I suggested she secretly disliked running. But the place we eventually arrived at in our conversation was a very honest one: Sheila was running out of punishment for having a body, and for having a body with fat. She didn't exercise because she loved movement. She ran because she hated weight. To my thinking, the intensely fearful thoughts that motivated her were causing a physiologic stress-response. This fight-or-flight state was exponentially increased by a form of exercise that didn't suit her body but in fact added even more stress chemistry. Running was not going to take her where she wanted to go and her weight was the proof.

Sheila understood this and agreed to completely drop all aspects of her marathon training. In place of running I asked her to choose something she would love to do. She decided to take a dance class three times per week and a yoga class three times per week and to do some occasional walking.

In three months' time Sheila lost the weight she had gained in the first weeks of her new diet, in addition to losing eight of the ten pounds she was originally hoping to lose. She was satisfied with her body, relieved that she didn't need to run like a hamster on a wheel, and was truly enjoying her newfound physical activity.

The moral of this story is not that exercise is bad. But we need to look at the motivating forces that drive us to exercise. Healthy habits driven by fear are not so healthy after all. Deep self-limiting thoughts can do nothing but suppress metabolism, even in the face of intense, calorie-burning workouts.

Can you see any implications for your own exercise style?

Week 6: Your Primary Task

This week is your opportunity to transform thoughts and feelings that suppress metabolism and limit happiness. Your primary task is to identify thoughts that drain energy and replace them with thoughts that gain energy. Think of week 6 as a new beginning in how you use your mind to support your highest intentions.

Exercise: Think Nutritionally

With pen and paper, take an inventory of the most common thoughts you repeat to yourself about eating, nutrition, and your body. These are the one-liners that together form your relationship with food and that ultimately help or hinder metabolism. Use the following questions to help guide you in your inventory. Be specific and thorough in your answers.

What do you tell yourself when you're eating?
What do you expect food to do for you?
What nutritional rules do you feel strongly about?
Which foods are on your "good" list?
Which foods constitute your "bad" list?
What are your rules about health, weight, and longevity?
What are your fears about health, weight, and longevity?
Is food your enemy or your ally, or is it a combination of the two?

Some examples of typical one-liners about food are these:

"Food makes me fat."
"Hunger is bad."
"I don't deserve to enjoy food."
"If I eat what I want, I won't be able to stop."
"Eating should make me happy and thin."
"These vitamins are good for me."
"Salt is bad for my blood pressure."
"Salads are healthy."
"Wine is good."
"Wine is bad."
"Any food containing fat is bad."

And so on.

Next, look over your list and put a check next to the thoughts that empower your metabolism and an X next to the ones that diminish it. A metabolically empowering thought encourages openness, possibility, and a joyous life experience. An energy-draining thought feels heavy and limiting and is designed to lead us into self-judgment.

Next, replace the energy-draining thoughts with metabolically inspiring ones. For example, if your thought was "Eating is a frustrating affair," your new thought might be "I am nourished by food." If your thought was "Food makes me fat," your new thought would be "I let go of my fears about weight." If your thought was "Ice cream is bad," your new thought could be "Ice cream is something I can either choose to eat or choose not to eat. Made wisely, either choice can support my metabolism."

Other positive and energy-enhancing thoughts include these: "I trust in the wisdom of my body"; "I welcome my desire for food"; "I let go of punishing myself for eating 'bad' foods"; and "I choose to relax about eating." Your job is to let new and inspiring thoughts abundantly inhabit your inner airwaves each day. Affirm these new thoughts as you eat. Repeat them to yourself before bed. Catch yourself when you think otherwise and compassionately make a correction within. In general, this week let go of all moralistic concepts of good food and bad food and allow the wisdom of your body to determine what is best for you.

Closely monitor your thoughts as you would the intake of food on a strict diet. And rather than let your thoughts think you, choose to claim the power to control your mental landscape. To the best of your ability, release all negative thinking about food, weight, and body. Stop the flow of toxic chemicals created by your inner pharmacy through fearful thoughts. Freedom and vitality will surely follow.

Exercise: Change Your Core Beliefs

Your next task is to identify and make a list of the core limiting beliefs you hold around food, body, health, and sexuality. This is an even deeper dive into how we think. It's about discovering the negative mantras that we silently and unknowingly speak to ourselves. These hidden mantras are the software programs that direct brain and body to construct a metabolic world of lack and limitation. Identifying and correcting them is a huge step in empowering the chemistry of the body. Here are some examples of core limiting beliefs.

"There is something wrong with my metabolism and I won't be happy until I fix it."

"I'll never be truly loveable unless I'm at my perfect weight."

"There's never enough for me in this world—never enough love, enough satisfaction, enough money, enough food."

"I didn't choose this body, these looks, or my life circumstances. I'm living the wrong life."

"There's not enough time to nourish myself. My body comes last."

"I can't let out my real passion and sexiness. I wouldn't be safe."

"I'm destined to have the same illness that my mother [or father] had."

"If I could only find the perfect diet, the perfect way to eat, then I'd be happy."

"The past is certain to repeat itself—I'm bound to be disappointed with weight-loss practices or in trying to improve my health."

"The world owes me. I haven't been given my due. People owe me, life owes me, God owes me."

"I'm a victim. The unhappy events in my life were done to me, against me. I've been wronged. None of it is my responsibility."

"I'm an imposter. I'm not good enough. I've got to pretend to be someone I'm not. If people knew the real me, I'd be totally alone."

How do you uncover your core limiting beliefs? It takes a little bit of soul-searching and a lot of self-honesty. Find some quiet time to reflect on the question: "What are the deepest fears that drive my life?" Your core limiting beliefs will come from answering this question. Sometimes a powerful question such as this needs to marinate for a few days. Listen to your dreams. Let the responses emerge into your awareness. You may find that you can clearly identify one core negative belief, or even a handful. Once you've identified them on paper, pull the plug on their power source by rescripting them into beliefs that elevate and inspire. Next to each negative belief write down its healthy opposite. If the old belief was "I'll never be truly loveable and attractive unless I'm at my perfect weight," your new core belief could be "I am loveable and desirable just as I am right now." If the old belief is "I'm living in the wrong body," its replacement could be "My body is the perfect vehicle for me to learn the lessons of love and to grow."

Repeat these new affirmations to yourself each day, reflect on them at night, tape them to your refrigerator or have someone close to you say them to you as often as possible. The transformation happens as you truly try on and absorb this new way of thinking and being. Success is in gentle, conscious, continuous effort throughout the week. If you catch yourself falling back in to the old belief, gracefully redirect the course of your thinking. This is a profound way to change your inner world, and thus the chemistry of the body.

Exercise: Inspiration Inventory

Take a moment to consider why you do what you do when it comes to your health. What motivates you to eat a good diet? To take vitamin supplements or medications? Why do you exercise? What forces are at work in your inner world that propel you to take action? Make a list of all the strategies you do during the course of the year that are intended to benefit your health. Then, next to each one, note whether you are motivated by fear or by love. Do you eat healthy because you love health or because you loathe disease? Are you exercising because you love movement and the feeling of fitness or because you despise body fat?

Next, consider the distinction between motivation and inspiration. Motivation, though a potentially positive attribute, is often used to push ourselves to act in ways that aren't truly resonant with our core values. People who say they're highly motivated are often highly stressed and physically drained from chasing after elusive goals. Inspiration, on the other hand, is a power that comes through us but is seemingly not of us. It is expansive, enlivening, limitless in supply, and leaves us metabolically enriched. How does inspiration register in your body? Does it give you a different metabolism?

During week 6, your task is to practice the eating principles you've been learning from a place of inspiration. Eat quality foods with relaxation, awareness, pleasure, and rhythm—not from a fear of fat or disease but from the love of living a healthy life. Perhaps the easiest way to feel inspiration is to invoke it. Ask it to enter in through your heart's doorway. Recall a time when you felt inspired to nourish yourself with good food and care for your body. What were the circumstances? Where did your inspiration come from? How did you maintain it? Visualize the you that was inspired, feel in your body what that inspired state felt like, and invite that inspired self into present time. From that place, make a list of anything you can do this week—especially the little things—that are inspirational for health. Practice them with gratitude and with a smile.

Exercise: A New Way to Move

Many of us approach fitness not so much out of love for exercise but as a reprimand for having body fat or eating food. Even though we may reap some of the benefits of exercise, our hidden world of fear and self-judgment will generate a metabolism that falls far short of its potential.

Similarly, many of us who choose not to exercise are also acting from a position of judgment and punishment. We abandon our bodies because of shame, grief, or the false belief that once we've let ourselves lose control of eating and exercise we can never recover. We secretly believe that we don't deserve better.

It's time to move closer to our own hearts and souls to examine what most often stops us—our fears—and to administer the proper medicine—compassion.

A useful distinction to proceed with is the difference between "movement" and "exercise." For many, exercise has the connotation of required, repetitive punishment. It's something we have to do as opposed to something we love to do. Movement is the antidote to exercise. It's a celebration of the body. It's inspired, it's natural, and it's born from a place of cellular joy. The same exercise, such as jogging or Stairmaster, can be done from love rather than punishment. It's all about our thinking.

In your journal, give thoughtful responses to these questions:

Do I exercise from a love of movement?

Are there any ways I use exercise as a punishment?

Have I abandoned my body when it comes to movement or exercise?

What are the specific judgments I have about my body?

Do these judgments serve me?

What stands in my way of inspired movement on a regular basis?

What would my life feel like if joyous, inspired movement was
regular fare?

What kind of movement or exercise would inspire me?

During week 6, transform the way you exercise. Move from a place of celebration. Make the commitment to find joy in your physicality. The specifics are simple: Observe your thoughts when you exercise. When you notice the inner critic is at the controls, gently invite in the compassionate and graceful dancer. In this way exercise, like eating, becomes a meditation in awareness. As with meals, breathe deeply and consciously as you move. This brings us into the present moment and into a more authentic relationship with the body. You needn't change the type of exercise you do. You simply need to change you, the exerciser.

Monitor yourself to see if you're receiving pleasure. Many people find that once they observe and release their negative mind-chatter about exercising, they have more energy, endurance, and a welcome lightness of body and being. For extra credit this week, choose a new way to move your body. Find an exercise or body discipline that's a departure from how you normally move. The choices these days are bountiful—Pilates, Gyrotonics, Feldenkrais, NIA. Think of this not as a replacement of your regular routine but an addition to it. If you're accustomed to aerobics, add some light weight training. If you're the type who focuses on competitive exercise, choose a more artful form of movement such as dance or tai chi. If you tend to go "hard"—doing heavy weights, intense aerobics, and so forth—try going "soft" with yoga, gentle stretching, swimming. Trust your body this week. Set it free to move. Ask your gut-intelligence for information about what your body wants, and listen for feedback in a deeper way than you ever have before.

The key to accessing the metabolic power of thinking is to become aware of your thoughts and then choose to change them. Observe your mind with persistence and patience. Affirm the energy-gaining thoughts and gently release the energy-draining ones. Discard all nutritional concepts that are rooted in judgment or fear. Invoke inspiration into your dietary world. Practice self-acceptance. And above all, believe in the power of belief to direct the course of your metabolic destiny in each and every moment.

Key Lessons

- What we think is electrochemically transduced into physiological responses.

- Thinking, therefore, is a nutritional choice.

- Negative thoughts about food can directly inhibit digestion through nerve pathways, hormones, neuropeptides, and other bio-substances. Positive thoughts about food enhance digestion via these same pathways.

- The placebo effect is proof positive that our thoughts, beliefs, and expectations can influence the metabolic effect of a food or supplement.

- The source of our motivation strongly influences metabolism. Healthy activities driven by fear can yield poor results, while the same action powered by inspiration can yield more positive results.

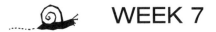 **WEEK 7**

The Metabolic Power of Story

The universe is made up of stories, not atoms.

MURIEL RUKEYSER, POET

Have you ever heard a story that inspired you or changed your life? One that lifted your spirits or gave you hope? The stories that move us are like powerful drugs that ignite our metabolism. There's a hidden narrator within each of us that puts a spin on every aspect of our journey. And that spin—whether it's positive and life affirming or negative and nihilistic—sets our metabolism in motion and creates a biochemistry that is a mirror image of our inner world. As we become more adept at discerning the secret stories we unwittingly tell, and as we're more willing to author a generous and healing tale, our metabolism rises according to the new standard we set.

Let's take a look at how we can harness the metabolic power of story.

The Story of DNA

If you consult with a doctor who cares about healing and knows what she or he is doing, the most important and telling part of the visit will be the taking of your history—your story. Who you are: the family you're born into; what you eat, drink, and dream; where you live; how you work and play; your relationships—every detail about you is a window into your metabolism. Your entire history is your story, and your story is everything.

Perhaps the most fundamental storybook found in the human library is our DNA.

At the molecular level, our genetic material tells a timeless and entertaining tale. The tale our DNA tells comes in twenty-three chapters, also known as chromosome pairs. The thirty thousand or so genes within the twenty-three chromosome chapters make up the subplots, characters, twists, and turns in our human book of life. Fortunately, there are multiple endings and possibilities in our genetic destiny because we choose so many of the variables that influence the expression of our genes—what we eat, how we exercise, where we reside, how we live and love.

If you believe in the science of genetics, then you believe that the phenomenon of story is built into the body and is the bottom-line reality of who we are. If Shakespeare was right (and I suspect he was) that indeed "the whole world is a stage," then the roles we play and the chemistry of who we are can only be one and the same. Like it or not, we're characters in a larger play and coauthors in the whole affair. The tales we weave are the foodstuff that fuels the body and animates our experience. Our story sits in the director's chair of each cell and organizes the molecular production crew to create the movie that is our life. The effects of story are felt from the densest level of biology to the most rarified atmosphere of the soul.

What I'm suggesting is this: DNA is nothing more than the biochemical equivalent of a story, and our personal story is the subtle equivalent of DNA. In other words, matter and energy are once again playfully exchanging their clothes. Fortunately, you don't have to rely on the mapping of the human genome to receive the benefits of genetic engineering. Changing your story is a much more safe and sane method for redirecting your DNA, and hence the course of your metabolism.

Who's Eating?

If you'd like to see the metabolic power of story in action, take a look at one of the most treasured possessions you have—your personality. Contrary to popular belief, neither you nor I can legitimately claim to be one person. Each of us is more like a crowd. We're each a collection of personalities and archetypes—mother, child, sister, lover, bitch, goddess, virgin, whore; father, son, brother, warrior, king, killer, victim, clown. The list, of course, is endless. Each of these characters has her or his own story, and each plays a part in service to the larger story of our life. Indeed, many psychologists are now suggesting that having multiple personalities, so to speak, is the most accurate model of how we truly function. In other words, the guy you call "me" is actually a bunch of different people, and who "me" is depends on who's home at the time.

Amazingly, researchers have discovered that, in patients with classic multiple personality disorder, each personality has a unique and distinct physiology.[1] Dramatic and measurable variations can be seen in heart rate, blood pressure, galvanic skin response, and hormone levels depending on which personality is predominant at the time. One individual was a clinically diagnosed insulin-dependent diabetic, but only in one specific personality. Another patient had a severe allergy to citrus fruits that would cause her to break out in hives, but again, only in one personality. The researcher could visually observe the hives disappearing as the patient made a switch to another persona.[2]

If it sounds far-fetched that each separate personality that populates such individuals has a different metabolism, consider how science has already elucidated the fact that every mode of consciousness—waking, sleeping, dreaming, stress, relaxation, and so on—has its own unique chemistry. Because we are biochemical beings, every cognitive state has its biochemical equivalent.

What the multiple personality patients teach us is that the story we live and the metabolism we experience are intricately linked. At any given meal, or in any given moment, one of the many characters that inhabit our inner sanctum sits at the head of the table. It has its own peculiar habits, its own quirky needs, and its unique nutritional metabolism.

Jeanette reports that she loves sponge cake but the sugar it contains sends her into a hypoglycemic response, so she avoids it altogether. When she visits her grandmother, though, sponge cake is always served, and it isn't a problem for her. During her childhood, grandma and sponge cake were one and the same, and the memories of those visits are most special for Jeanette. Could it be that her "granddaughter personality" has a healthier blood-sugar regulation?

Sarah, a business consultant, remarked "I've got two stomachs—a kosher one and a nonkosher one. At home I strictly follow Jewish dietary law. If I eat a nonkosher food in my apartment I feel absolutely nauseous and sick. But during business luncheons I don't always have the luxury of keeping kosher, so something inside me takes over and I can handle any food without a problem."

The important question here is this.

When you sit down to a meal, who is eating?

Jack, a twenty-nine-year-old engineer, complained about poor digestion, heartburn, and an inability to lose weight. He had a family history of diabetes and cardiovascular disease, so losing fifteen pounds was a priority. The problem was, Jack had no willpower. He'd eat right for several days, at which time his digestion would feel fine. But then he'd lapse into a high cream cheese, high potato chip, low vegetable diet, at which point he'd experience intense gastric upset. Jack's methodical engineer's mind couldn't figure out why he would eat against his own wishes.

I saw that some part of Jack was clearly getting in his own way and suggested that for several weeks, before beginning any meal or snack, he ask himself one simple question: "Who's eating?" I explained the possibility that different archetypal characters people our inner world and that it might serve Jack well to identify exactly who was at the table at any given moment in time. I requested that he not fight any of these voices, that he not judge them or overpower them or change them in any way. He just needed to observe and gather information.

Jack was both amused and intrigued. He took the advice to heart and here's what he discovered: "When I checked in to see who was eating, I saw that the rebel in me is always there when I'm breaking the rules, and it's the rebel that gets heartburn. It takes over whenever anyone tries to boss me around or give me rules to live by. I always thought I had no willpower with food but I really do—it's inside my rebel. I just needed to find a way for that will to work for me, not against me."

In a short period of time Jack learned to listen to his inner rebel, to dialogue with it and understand it and accept it, and to give the rebel what it needed so that Jack could have what he needed. As long as Jack let the rebel break a rule once or twice a week, everyone was happy. He saw that it was the rebel who actually supplied him with his strength and his feisty nature. His digestive issues significantly cleared within weeks and his weight dropped slowly over the course of the next four months.

Think about some of the many personalities you have—the different faces you adopt around friends and family, at work and on vacation, and the hidden sides of you that emerge when circumstances are just right. How do these personalities differ in their choice of foods? Are there noticeable changes in your body when you're in certain personas? Do you notice changes in digestion?

Can you see how the phenomenon of multiple personalities might affect your everyday metabolism?

What's Your Story?

Luccia, thirty-five, a mother of two, was having trouble losing weight. She also had chronic headaches and worsening allergies. Like many savvy and dedicated people I encounter, she'd tried a number of traditional and holistic strategies without success. A highly educated and skilled special-education teacher, Luccia was now devoting all of her time to family. It didn't take long to see that she was living the life of a martyr. Her daily schedule was all about cooking meals, cleaning up, chauffeuring kids, snacking them, attending to her husband before and after work, and visiting her elderly mother. Luccia would never sit down to eat, nor would she prepare her own meal. She scavenged for leftovers from her kids' plates, eating arrhythmically and under stress with no pleasure, no awareness—the usual American way.

As she spoke more about her home life and her inner world, a hidden story line emerged. Luccia was subservient to men and she felt inferior to the males in her life. She was raised in the Midwest but her husband was from another culture, one that traditionally expected women to do everything. She would silently take on his backward demands with a manner and a smile that was inconsistent with the violation she was truly feeling. Her fourteen-year-old son had assumed the habits of his dad and did nothing around the home to help. The son she loved was growing up to be the kind of man who made her feel small and inconsequential.

For Luccia, diets didn't work, exercise failed, and drugs only masked her symptoms because of one reason: Her story was toxic. Her core beliefs were: "I don't count. My needs come last. Men are my superiors. That's my lot in life, so I have to bury all my feelings of pain and protest and take things with a fake smile." This tale was placing the burden of a physiologic stress-response on her metabolism, which in turn impaired her digestion and her ability to burn calories and helped cause her headaches.

As we spoke, Luccia was relieved and tearful to have a man honor and acknowledge her story of wounding. She quickly and intuitively recognized the connections between the problems in her body and the way she authored her life story. I suggested the key change she needed to make was to start believing she mattered, that she was equal alongside men, and to act as if it were so. From this new place, we devised some simple actions she could take: enroll her son in cooking, cleaning, and taking care of his younger sister; have her husband make his own breakfast and pack his own lunch; and have one evening each week set aside for dinner and a date at a restaurant of her choosing, a standing date each week when her husband gets to treat her like a queen.

What might sound like mundane strategies were instead deeply meaningful. Luccia was helping to rewrite not only her own story but those of her immediate family and perhaps even the stories of the generations before her who helped pass these tales down. Within a few months Luccia lost the handful of pounds that was burdening her and her digestive issues and headaches were down to a minimum. Her body had less weight because her story had lightened up.

Can you see how underneath every possible issue we face with food, health, or weight is a story that shapes our metabolic reality?

Re-storying is not only a radical act of self-respect, it's also a powerful form of self-initiation. In high school and college, someone else decides when you're qualified to graduate. In the school of life, you've got the ultimate say. Self-graduation means you decide when it's time to elevate yourself. You choose to become the playwright of your journey and to craft a tale that's true to the heart.

Indeed, whatever spin we put on our story—happy, hopeful, paranoid, positive—is the precise way our molecules spin into motion and embody those qualities at the cellular level. It's no accident that molecular physicists describe subatomic particles as having charm and personality. Put a negative spin on your story about health, weight, food, exercise, or life and the exact conditions are in place to deplete the body and age it in fast-forward. That's because negativity creates a physiologic stress-response, which means oxygen depletion, free-radical formation, and the production of chemicals that are inflammatory, mutagenic, autoimmune, and cytotoxic. Put a positive spin on your personal fable and you create the chemistry of relaxation and pleasure, which catalyzes oxygenation, circulation, immunity, nutrient assimilation, calorie burning, and cellular regeneration. The science is simple and straightforward.

It's fascinating how our culture elevates its stories to lofty and honorable heights—think of *The Wizard of Oz, Gone with the Wind, Lord of the Rings*—yet when it comes to the business of scientific research and discovery, story takes a backseat. What I mean is this: The validity of a medical study is founded upon its success in pulling out the intangibles, the invisibles, the richness, and flattening out all variables so we can test one drug or nutrient against a theoretically homogenous population. We pull out the story. That's why the ultimate insult one scientist can hurl at another is "Your evidence is anecdotal." That is, "There's no real proof. All you have is just a bunch of stories."

And yet, all there is is story. Life is a story. And science is but one story about the world. When we finally get down to the business of how the body truly works, story will be seen for what it is—the highest form of proof, not the lowest. We've allowed ourselves to plunge so deep into the mechanistic story of things that the magic of the world has retreated. If you don't live in an enchanted body, how bright do you think your metabolic fire can be? Indeed, our inner flame is sparked to life by the friction created when the storied life of the soul courses through the pathways of the body—its nerves, vessels, sinews, and cells. Allow the richest imaginings of the soul to take root within and our metabolism is given the most vital nutrients it will ever need.

A New Nutritional Beginning

Have you ever had the experience of looking out an airplane window and suddenly seeing your life from a higher perspective? The hectic world that engulfed you moments ago now seems so small in the context of more important things. The expansive view removed you a bit, softened some hard edges, and allowed for deeper insights to emerge. Well, no matter what story you're living out with food and health, I'd like to suggest a way to borrow from such an experience to gain a fresh perspective, wipe your slate clean, and revitalize your metabolism. To do so, we need to view the body and its nourishment from the highest possible vantage point.

The trick I've discovered is to take all the known facts about food and nutritional metabolism, all the dietary wisdom on the planet, every piece of information on the subject you can possibly imagine, every book and every study, and sum it all up into a one-sentence story that says it all. Sounds impossible?

Well, I believe I've got it figured out—the mother of all nutrition stories condensed into one line. Check it out and see what you think:

You're born, you eat, you die.

That's it. That's the bottom line and the ultimate test and proof of any diet—be it high protein, low fat, paleo, vegetarian, raw food, junk food, or any other approach under the sun. As far as the scientific community can tell, and according to mere anecdotal evidence, we're all destined for the same fate no matter how perfect our diet or how tight our abs. I'm not saying all this out of a morbid desire to ruin your day but because such knowledge has the power to liberate us. So much of our energy is secretly channeled into strategies for cheating death and preventing the eventual demise of the body. But if we can begin to accept our final destiny now, then our journey can proceed with more merriment and mirth and we can create the fertile conditions for the kind of metabolism we wish to express during our Earthly visit.

With the final end in mind—"you die"—and with the unchangeable start of our nutritional journey—"you're born"—what we're left with in the "you eat" portion of life's program is a big choice. It's a blank slate. A clean page. You make up the story. You choose the plot. Each of us has nutritional free will. In the "you eat" phase of your existence, there are no rules other than the ones you and I invent. Isn't it great that we're given so much room to create? So the point is, we'd be doing ourselves a wonderful favor to ask the question "What's the purpose of eating the way I eat?"

Indeed, there are plenty of people who will tell you, "Hey, I'm going to die anyway so I might as well eat whatever I want and enjoy it." Quite frankly, that's a perfectly valid choice as long as it's consciously chosen and coming from a place of responsibility and empowerment. Some people who say this really mean it and are quite happy, while others secretly want to take better care of themselves but have no available tools to help release themselves from self-punishment and abuse.

At another end of the spectrum, we have the power to choose a style of eating that is infused with deeper meaning. Indeed, one of the more thoughtful ways we can evolve our relationship with food, and hence our metabolism, is to align our way of eating with our greater life purpose. That means getting in touch with the story of who we are and why we're here on Earth, and eating in a way that supports this grander mission.

Mission statements are pretty popular these days. Just about any business you do commerce with has spent time, energy, and money to articulate its larger purpose so that the people behind the business can be certain of who they are, can function with efficiency, and can court success. What I'm suggesting is that if Burger King and Jack-in-the-Box can have a mission statement, so can you and I.

See if you can write down in three sentences or less the essence of your mission on planet Earth. It might be helpful to voice your purpose first in the most general terms, with statements such as "I'm here to raise my children and care for my loved ones"; "I'm here to share my love with the world"; "I'm here to contribute my talents to leave behind a better place." You can also get as specific as you'd like, such as "I'm here to help others heal"; "I'm here to help educate young people and give them a positive start"; "I'm here to help people invest their money, create wealth, and support good causes."

Whatever mission statement you choose for now, I suggest you proceed to view your diet, exercise, and the nourishment of your body in the context of that mission. In other words, what manner and style of eating would help you if your mission was to make an important contribution to your family and loved ones? Well, it would at least need to be a nutritional approach that kept you happy, healthy, and well fed so you could continue to give your best. If your life's mission is focused on work and career, you'd probably want the kind of relationship with food that is flexible enough to fit your work style yet keeps your mind clear and your body feeling energized and light. If your mission includes somehow leaving the world a better place, then you'd likely choose a way of eating that is supportive of the Earth, its soil, and all the creatures in its care.

So take a look at your mission statement and create a list in your journal of all the specific details and general attributes of how your eating day would unfold if it were in alignment with and in service to your higher purpose. Once you've got this down on paper, you'll have a guiding star by which to steer your metabolism. It will be easier to work with yourself rather than against yourself. Yes, there is plenty of room for your more personal and self-focused desires—a leaner body and a sexier physique. But now you can move from a more soulful perspective because you'll be putting first things first. In doing so you might find that some of the charge you've experienced around attaining metabolic perfection is diffused. Paradoxically, this release of a fear-driven focus will free up your metabolism and allow it to naturally reach a higher place. After all, how can you possibly lose weight if you can't lighten up? And how can you expect to increase the heat of your metabolic fire if you keep dampening it with a flood of fears?

A Happy Dietary Ending

Another important way to maximize the metabolic power of story is to invent for yourself a happy dietary ending. Better still, I'd like to share with you a way that can almost guarantee such an outcome. Here's the process.

First, make a list of all the benefits you expect to receive once you've reached your goals with eating, weight, energy, fitness, and health. In other words, why would you want to eat better? Why do you want to lose weight? Why would you want a different shape? More energy? Greater health? Take a moment to write down all the benefits you anticipate will be yours once you've arrived at your desired destination. Some of the typical benefits people expect from having a healthier metabolism include "I'll have more energy"; "I'll feel better about myself"; "I'll feel lighter"; "I'll fit into my clothes"; "I'll be more attractive and desirable"; "I'll be more confident"; "I'll finally be the person who I really am"; "I'll accomplish more"; "I'll have a better experience of life."

Now here's the trick to assuring your happy ending:

Whatever benefits you expect to be yours at the end of your dietary efforts, simply receive them in the beginning.

If you think you'll be happy once you lose ten pounds, be happy now. If you imagine you'll have more energy when you finally eat right, have more energy now. If you believe you'll be more confident and loveable when you have the body you want, be more confident and loveable now. Whatever benefits you expect at the end, generate them in the beginning. Take on that personality, that role, that story. Act as if you already are the person you wish to be. We worship the stars and starlets of Hollywood for their ability to make us believe in the stories and characters they portray. It's a fabulous talent that, behold, you and I are well endowed with. Act as if you are the person you wish to be and you'll not only convince the rest of us but you'll also prove it to yourself. You'll literally generate the physiology of the character you're portraying—the metabolic power of story is that potent and real.

If you look over the list of benefits you expect to receive, you'll notice that almost all of them are a choice you can make in this instant. Indeed, perhaps the ultimate benefit of any diet or fitness program, the one that supercedes them all, is that we'll be happier. Why wait? Choose to be happier now, act more energetic and light now, be more sexy now, act healthier now and you'll already be at your final destination. And magically, by self-generating the end results in the beginning, you'll create the precise metabolic environment for those benefits to truly materialize and take hold even more.

You'll have cultivated the chemistry of relaxation, pleasure, deeper oxygenation, awareness, empowered thought, and aligned rhythm, all of which fan our metabolic flames. Whatever chemistry we create along our journey informs the chemical conclusion we reach at the end. Do you really believe that weight loss will come any easier if you're living out a story that produces the physiology of self-judgment and negativity? Do you honestly imagine that the right nutritional approach will grant you more energy if the story you live along the way continues to drain it? Even in the worst-case scenario, if you choose to be happy at the beginning and you don't lose the weight you wanted to lose, at least you'll still be happy.

It only takes a moment for metabolism to rearrange itself in response to our story. Recall a time when you were feeling low energy or low metabolism and an unexpected visitor or phone call instantly lifted your spirits. That person or message had a certain meaning for you, put a positive and inspiring spin on your story of the moment, which in turn spun your subatomic particles in just the right way to activate your inner feel-good pharmacy. We can invoke this same metabolic magic by rewriting our stories in any given moment and bringing the happy ending we've always hoped for into present time.

Week 7: Your Primary Task

This week is your opportunity to reflect upon how you author your relationship to food and hence how you author the chemistry of the body. This is your chance to do a surgical strike on the storylines that fail to serve and to leave in their place a healthier and more vibrant tale. Your primary task is to identify your nutritional story, recast it in a higher light, and experience the results.

Exercise: Your Metabolic History

We begin week 7 with your most substantive journaling exercise of the Slow Down program. Your assignment is to write down your complete food, diet, and body history. Consider this to be a thorough biography from infancy to the present day of your personal metabolic journey. Do this exercise when you have at least an hour of quiet, undisturbed time. Be considerate with yourself as you recount sweet memories, difficult ones, and as you tell an accurate and honest tale. Write down whatever flows through you without editing as you go or trying to get it "right." Here are some guidelines to help you in this process.

- Describe the various diets, nutritional systems, and approaches to food you've taken since childhood and throughout life.
- List the nutrition and diet beliefs you've felt most strongly about and the changes those beliefs have undergone.
- Describe your important life experiences with health, energy level, and disease. What have been your biggest challenges in these areas? Your successes? How did illnesses, accidents, or time spent in recovery impact your personal and inner worlds?
- Describe your relationship to your body—and your body image—from childhood to the present.
- Describe your experiences of sexuality and sensuality from childhood to the present. What were your biggest challenges? Breakthroughs? Note any connections between these and your relationship to food and body image.
- How have parents, friends, relatives, and partners influenced and affected your experience of food, health and body throughout the years?
- Have you ever felt betrayed around your health or body? How does this influence you today?
- What are the secrets around food, health, and body that you keep most concealed? What are your biggest fears? How do these secrets or fears affect you?
- What are your most positive and inspiring memories with food, health, sexuality, and your body? When was (or will be) the "prime of your life" in these areas? When have you felt the most vitality? What were your most significant breakthroughs with food?

When you're finished, take some time to reread and absorb what you've written. This is a powerful document. Be present with yourself and with any feelings that may have come up. Write down any new insights that may have arisen during this process or any connections that you might have made. Are there any themes that stand out for you? Can you identify more clearly the core beliefs that influenced your metabolic past? Do you see any attributes of your character you'd like to change?

Oftentimes what stops us from letting go of unwanted habits in the present is how we interpret our story from the past. Hidden beneath the radar of our conscious awareness, we carry tales from another time that burden us with their weight. And the more we try to escape our unredeemed past, the more it holds us in an invisible grip.

Once you've sat with your metabolic history—your old nutritional story—and absorbed its meaning in your life, it's time to look at the past through fresh eyes.

Exercise: Rewrite Your Nutritional Past

Now go back to the themes, the storylines, you've uncovered in writing in your metabolic history and do a brave, creative edit. How can you spin your tale so it's a wholly positive one? How can you reinterpret your story so that all the seeming setbacks, abandonments, hardships, illnesses, weight issues, diet challenges, and uncertainties are seen as the perfect journey you needed to take to learn the lessons most important for your soul's growth? Can you instill love in your story? Can you author a belief in the goodness of people, including yourself? Can you find forgiveness? A peaceful acceptance of what is? Consider this exercise as an opportunity to make peace with an important part of yourself.

Rewriting your nutritional history and casting it in the wise and compassionate light of the soul is a powerful means of liberating energy and healing our most persistent ailments and wounds. Once you've created your new and wholly positive tale about your nutritional past, take some time to reread and absorb it. Visit it throughout the week to remind yourself of the true story of your bodily life—a story written from the wisdom of love.

Have you ever met someone who has had a dramatic turnaround in her or his health or weight? Someone who became "born again" in his or her body and is now more vibrantly alive, radiant, happy, and inspired? Do you honestly think such a transformation could be merely the result of lower calorie meals, more mileage on the treadmill, or a feel-good supplement?

I'm willing to bet large sums of cash that regardless of the nutritional program, fitness system, or exercise gizmo that person employed, what really fueled the fires of his or her metabolic rebirth was a new story. You could put anybody on the best diet in the galaxy, but if that person is living in fear and motivated by a pessimistic plot, then the benefits of all her or his good work will never fully take hold.

Exercise: Your New Nutritional Story

Your next task is to create a whole new nutritional story that takes you from this moment into the future. This is your opportunity to begin your relationship with food anew. It's your chance to design the direction of your dietary life from the deepest level, and in doing so, to impact the quality of your biochemistry for years to come.

In your journal, screen-write the movie about food, body, health, and sexuality that you'll be acting the central part in for the rest of your life. Create an inspiring story that you'd be charmed to live in. What will you eat? How will you nourish yourself? Where will you eat? With whom? How will you feel? How will your body feel? How will you nourish others? What will be your experience of pleasure? How will you delight yourself? How will you take responsibility for the Earth? The plants? The animals? The hungry ones? What will be your main philosophy about food and health? What specific principles will you choose to believe and act upon? How will your mornings look different? Your conversations? How will you exercise and move? Will you look in the mirror with new eyes? Will you honor yourself? What will the last chapter of your nourishment story say? Refer to the mission statement on page 150. See how it fits into your new story. Also, refer back to the section "A Happy Dietary Ending" on pages 151–153. Again, see how you can integrate this approach, always keeping the end goal of all your dietary efforts in mind at the beginning. Write down in as much detail as possible your new life themes. Then, for the remainder of week 7 and beyond, live out this new story.

It might be helpful to make a list of the practical ways you can begin to enact your new tale. Each day this week, revisit what you've written to remind yourself of your new story. Enjoy this fresh start. Believe in it. Believe in yourself. Enlist friends and loved ones to support you in your new role. If you're not sure where to focus first, do what inspires you the most. And notice the results in body and being of your new nutritional story.

Exercise: Who's Eating?

Here's a final and fun exercise for week 7. Whenever you sit down to meals or snacks, ask yourself "Who's eating?" Amuse yourself with the task of identifying the particular subpersonality who is currently in charge and ready to eat. Some of the common characters who show up at the table include the rebel, the little girl or boy, the victim, the judge, the wolf, the saboteur, the perfectionist, the pleasure seeker, and the teenager. There are certainly plenty more. With just a little self-honesty, you'll find it quite easy to name the inner character who is speaking the loudest and wanting satisfaction.

Once you identify a subpersonality, dialogue with it and befriend it. Ask it what it wants. Why is this character present? Have you been neglecting her? Does she have a message for you? What bargain might you strike to satisfy some of her needs, yet still take care of the most important requirements of the health and happiness of the whole crew? Do your best to kindly understand this voice, learn the lessons it teaches, and receive the gifts it can give. If you're the kind of person who feels challenged by bouts of overeating or junk-food bingeing, try this strategy: invite your inner adult to the table more consistently. Many people think they need to contact their inner child, but I've noticed that when it comes to food, the inner child receives plenty of airtime. See how your inner woman or inner man can participate in the nourishment process. Notice how this adult character can readily assist you in enlightened eating choices and is happy to help.

The simple act of asking "Who's eating?" and witnessing who is truly present and metabolizing at each meal enables us to better feed the parts we'd like to nourish most. It's a rich and rewarding dialogue with the invisible characters who truly people our private universe. Ultimately, no one shows up to eat unless you send them an invitation. Are you ready to take full charge of your guest list?

Key Lessons

- Our inner story holds important keys to unlocking our metabolic power.

- By rewriting our story we can literally transform health, improve digestion, and enhance calorie-burning capacity.

- Each time we eat, a specific personality or archetypal character sits at the head of our inner table. The identity of that character will greatly determine our eating experience and the metabolism of our meal. We have the power to choose "who eats."

- Acknowledge your grander mission in life and allow your relationship with food to serve that mission.

- Whatever benefits you expect to receive at the end of a diet, create and experience those benefits in the beginning.

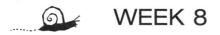 WEEK 8

The Metabolic Power of the Sacred

We are lived by powers we pretend to understand.

W. H. AUDEN

Have you ever had a religious, divine, or extraordinary experience that affected you deeply? One that left you feeling renewed, reborn, transformed in body or spirit? One that couldn't be explained, yet you know it happened? If so, then you surely experienced the metabolic power of the sacred.

Because each of us is a radiant soul moving through life's journey in a biological spacesuit, every soul experience is registered within as a metabolic event. We experience the world because chemistry helps make it so. Our feelings of love, for example, owe their existence to a specific chemistry generated in the body that is unique and specific to love. The same is true for feelings of hope, loyalty, silliness, cynicism, and any imaginable personality state. Who we are and what we feel moment to moment has a precise biochemical equivalent.

Sacred metabolism is the chemistry ignited in the body when we are infused by the Divine. Because the Divine is the source of power behind all powers, the chemistry created when we experience the Divine supercedes all known laws of the body. Sacred chemistry is a meta-chemistry. Its effects can include or incorporate familiar psycho-physiologic states such as the relaxation response, brain-hemispheric synchronization, pleasure chemistry, immune-system mobilization, and others. But certainly its boundaries far surpass what science can explain. When we enter the realm of sacred metabolism, then, we are on new scientific ground. The most reliable tools we have to proceed with are observation, experience, and the light of the truth.

Some of the ways that sacred metabolism may be revealed in the body include prayer, fasting, meditation, experiences in nature, sports, yoga, music, dance, a sweat lodge, artistic pursuits, sleeplessness, illness, recovery, near-death experiences, transformational drugs, sexual intimacy, stressful events, war, injury, hunting, grief, falling in love, and religious rituals of every variety.

When the metabolic power of the sacred is activated in the body, a portal is opened to a fantastic assortment of biological empowerments that would otherwise have no entry point. History is replete with examples of saints, yogis, shamans, messiahs, and ordinary folk whose fantastic metabolic powers are legendary. An abundance of well-documented cases have highlighted abilities such as clairvoyance, telekinesis, spontaneous healing, incredible strength, and the mystifying intellectual capacities of savants, to name just a few. But what we oftentimes label as anomalous or miraculous are simply latent biological traits activated once we are touched by the hand of the Divine.

Where this leaves us, of course, is at the frontier. Most of what we know about the capabilities of the human form is but the tiniest fraction of what is possible. Could it be that the advances in well-being that medical science has promised for decades, but still longs to deliver, will come not from anything outside of us—experts and technology—but will arrive through our coevolutionary relationship with the Divine? Is it possible that the fulfillment of your metabolic destiny is to be found inside you, intelligently seeded there and awaiting your discovery?

Eight Sacred Metabolizers

The question that's certainly worth asking is this: How can we engage the metabolic power of the sacred? In what ways can we reliably court its powers? Many believe the answer is austere religious practices or intense hours of yoga or meditation. But I would suggest that the sacred has its own terms that are available to all in this time and place, and those terms are these: love, truth, courage, commitment, compassion, forgiveness, faith, and surrender.

These eight sacred metabolizers—and no doubt there are more— are sacred because such soul qualities bring us closer to the heart of the Divine, to the intelligence that created us. By embodying them we become more like the source from whence we came, more of who we are meant to be and who we know, somewhere inside, we want to be. And I'm suggesting that when activated in our system, the eight sacred metabolizers can produce profound healings and powers, metabolic breakthroughs, and rejuvenating effects on body and spirit.

Essentially, these eight metabolizers have been classically viewed as qualities or traits, not material quantities unto themselves. And yet I would say that every sacred metabolizer is both a force and a substance. $E = MC^2$. Somewhere in the body, love molecules squirt about when feelings of love are activated. Perhaps it's a class of chemicals, or maybe there's a central love molecule around which the others gather and carouse. Similarly, when feeling courage the body will create the chemical equivalent of that trait in order for you and I to experience it. That's the nature of reality as it is lived in the biology of a body. Every feeling has a molecular correlate. Such substances arise in response to the soul invoking those qualities. First comes the thought or feeling, then comes the molecule.

Right now, think of someone in your life who pushes your buttons or stresses you out. If you focus hard enough on that person's faults, you'll phone in an order to your inner pharmacy and quickly fill a prescription for stress chemicals to be delivered throughout the body. We create our chemistry instantaneously, as fast or faster than the speed of light. And just as the biblical God proclaimed "Let there be light" and it was created, so too do we create ourselves moment to moment. When you say "Let there be anger," the body instantly builds a universe of anger within. When we say "Let there be kindness," kindness chemistry is fashioned in a like manner.

We are that powerful.

Observe your own life and you'll probably notice that the larger life we live in has its brilliant way of evoking the sacred eight—love, truth, courage, compassion, commitment, forgiveness, faith, surrender. They're often at center stage of our most important life passages and lessons. The more our soul yearns for these qualities and the more we call them forth and create them through our personal efforts, the more these molecules literally build in our system and work their metabolic magic. If that sounds far-fetched to you, consider that this concept is no different from Prozac. You take a bunch of pills that were produced in an outside chemical factory (as opposed to your internal one), and the critical molecules need to build in your system for weeks until they lift your spirits, so to speak.

Likewise, the more faith you have, or the more you exercise faith, the more faith molecules accumulate and build in your bloodstream. The metabolic substance of faith activates core organ systems such as the heart and brain and exerts its effects throughout the body—effects as simple as invigorating and healing or as profound as releasing the Mother Teresa or the Martin Luther King Jr. within.

Because the eight sacred metabolizers are experiences, they are "felt" within the body. For the purposes of discussion we can therefore call them "feelings." And like any feelings, the only way they can be felt is if we feel them. Strangely enough, many of us experience these feelings, but only in partial form. We have faith—sometimes, maybe. We love—but only so far. We're compassionate—but only toward a chosen few. And we call upon courage—but we shy away from it when facing our greatest fears. Whenever we feel such feelings partially, we undernourish the soul and literally rob the body of nutrition. We limit the circulation of the cosmic force of life and suppress metabolism. Conversely, the deeper we feel our feelings, the more we expand into our metabolic potential and the closer we come to the Divine.

Just as exercise puts a demand on the body to build more muscle, utilize oxygen more efficiently, and increase our capacity to breathe, so too does the simple act of being alive as a soul on planet Earth place the "demand" upon us to act with more faith, build more commitment, and live in greater truth. Life itself is the proper fitness regime. The eight sacred metabolizers are as essential to the body as food and water and are literally required in chemical form. If the soul craves love, then so does the body. If the soul craves the lessons of forgiveness, then our cells yearn for those molecules. If life is calling us to compassion, then this nutrient is required for our growth and repair. If you're alive and breathing, the divine realms are calling upon you to produce the chemistry that would elevate you to your highest metabolic potential via the soul lessons that will forge your greatest spiritual strength.

So if you think your nutritional concerns can be rightfully addressed with food alone, think again. When the real-life requirements of the eight sacred metabolizers are not met, the body withers and weakens, loses integrity, and invites disease upon itself, calling forth whatever symptoms are necessary to alert us to the soul lesson that is hungering for nourishment and attention. We can no longer look exclusively in the biological realm to solve health problems that are but downstream effects of the affairs and tides of the soul.

This is not an antiscientific stance. It is preeminently proscience, a call to allow the language of the soul, and of the sacred, back into the halls of medicine from whence it has been cast out. It's high time that we acknowledge the reality of the Divine no matter what our religious beliefs and invite the sacred to inform our practices of healing, eating, loving, and all our earthly pursuits.

Phil, a fifty-two-year-old computer-company executive, came to see me for weight loss. He was 6'3", a soft-spoken, sweet, gentle giant of a man who'd gained almost forty pounds in one year and couldn't take that weight off. Phil was a deeply caring being who took pride in building strong relationships with the people he managed. His company was going through reorganization and massive layoffs, and he was quite concerned for his staff. Phil admitted that he wasn't very motivated to lose weight even though his doctors had sounded off numerous alarms. He had tried a number of diets and seen a dietician but he couldn't stick to any program. He was perplexed because he considered himself a strongly motivated man, but in this particular area he had no willpower. Phil knew something was in his way but he couldn't figure out what that was, so he came to see me for "motivation."

It was clear to me that Phil was troubled about something deeper, and when I questioned him about the onset of his weight gain he conceded it was coincident with some personal issues at home that were difficult for him to discuss. His son was sent to prison for five years without parole for selling marijuana. It was a terrible shock for everyone, including Phil, whose world had come crashing down. His son was finishing college when he was arrested; he was an excellent student, responsible and popular. He had a great life in front of him. He never imagined he'd get caught selling pot. Phil was ashamed—he felt that he was a failure as a father and he felt helpless to change the situation and frightened for the well-being of his son, who was obviously not the type to fare well in prison life (as if there is such a person).

Phil was face to face with the greatest existential challenge of his life. Having his son in prison made no sense to him. It was hurling him into a search for meaning and for greater understanding. Phil didn't like religion, yet he found himself asking questions and looking for hope in places he previously had little interest in visiting. Given this opening, I suggested he would find his motivation to lose weight once he found some kind of faith. His metabolic concerns would be handled when he finally believed there was a higher wisdom to life and a greater plan for his son that was somehow the right soul medicine for everyone involved. Once he believed in something more, and stayed grounded there, he could trust that his son was guided and protected. And with that in place, he could forgive the party who he felt should bear the most guilt—himself.

Phil's weight was really a hidden cure. It was the remedy for his self-punishment, guilt, powerlessness, and, ultimately, his disconnection from the Divine. His forty extra pounds represented an abundant supply of stored energy. That's all excess body fat is, according to traditional science, and it's true—fat is stored energy. Yet for Phil this stored energy was more than a bunch of calories to fuel his exercise. It would be the fuel for a new life, a new relationship to the Divine, and a new journey with his son.

True to his nature, Phil's motivated self returned, and he made the switch to a new story that connected him to the sacred. Interestingly, Phil decided he didn't want me to provide any dietary advice for losing the weight—he was now confident in his own insights and didn't want to be disturbed by anyone else's methods. He eventually lost thirty of the forty pounds he'd gained. Once at this plateau, he chose to exert no further effort and would gladly bear the remaining weight until his son was released from prison. That's what felt right to him, that's how he scripted it, and that's what gave him some needed inspiration. By accessing the sacred metabolic powers of trust, faith, and forgiveness, Phil enabled himself to lose weight by gaining a personal connection to the cosmos.

Take a moment to consider the times in life when you were called upon to show up with a higher love, more compassion, greater courage or trust, a more steadfast commitment, deeper forgiveness, and a more encompassing faith, or a time when you were called upon to speak a more powerful truth. How did these experiences change your life? Did they affect your body? Your health? Your energy level? Did they leave you with a permanent and discernable metabolic gift? How can you invoke these qualities so their healing powers can be more consistently available in your life?

Nutrition Lessons for the Soul

By now I hope you're beginning to see that every issue or challenge we face with food and nutrition has a deep spiritual component. Of course, it's useful and necessary to address our metabolic concerns with the tools of medicine and science. But to truly transform and heal the ailments of the body, the soul perspective needs to be understood. For this reason, I'd like to suggest a way to view metabolism from the vantage point of the sacred. It's a radical rewrite of how we view the body. Our reigning story about health is that disease is bad: it's the enemy, the problem, and the poison. Any unwanted symptom—excess weight, low energy, digestive pains, and the like—are squarely seen as our adversary.

Allow me to propose the exact opposite:

Whatever you believe is the disease is actually the cure.
Whatever bodily concern you believe is the problem
is, in the soul's reality, the solution.

I know this may sound a bit strange to some, so let me elaborate. To the ancient Greeks, every symptom was seen as a visitation from the gods. Whatever afflicted the body was divine, a holy messenger, a whispered secret from the guardian spirits alerting us that the soul was in need of a course correction. The ailments of the body were really cures for the soul. And whatever cured the soul was the fundamental and necessary medicine for the body. By addressing the symptoms—listening to them, honoring them, being with them, welcoming their divinity—the soul would find its way through the mists, and the grey clouds raining poison on the body would lift.

Let's take a look at low energy, for example. What could it possibly be a cure for? What messages can lethargy and fatigue bring, and how would it be a blessing from the gods that could cure an ailment in the soul and thus complete the sacred circle and bring restoration back to the body? Well, interestingly enough, any disorder that brings us low energy is often the only way to slow us down. Speed is the disease. Low energy is the cure. It's a remedy for when we aren't attending to our deeper needs, when we're lost in the business of doing and forgetting how to simply be and feel.

Like it or not, low energy brings us into compliance with the slower pace of the soul. It's mandatory meditation, a forced vacation. It urges us to discover where our energy leakages are and where our life truly wants to go. Find the messages the gods are delivering through this ailment and you've found a cure for your life and for the body that was kind enough to slow you down and bring you home. Are you feeling low energy because there's merely something wrong with your body, or are you needing to be in touch with the reality that you work hard and require rest? Even God rested after six days of creative work. Do you think you've got a better system?

No matter what the cause, whatever we consider the disease is still the cure. Even if your fatigue is catalyzed by a food allergy, the wrong diet, a parasite, or poor sleep, you can only find the remedy to restore your body to health once you slow down, pay attention, care for yourself, look for help, and explore. It matters little to the soul what mechanism it employs to alert us to its calling.

And what would you imagine excess weight to be a cure for? For many, it's a wake-up call for a life out of balance. It asks us to look at our relationship to the earth, to each other, and to ourselves. Obesity is not the highly personal issue it's cracked up to be. Yes, it is personal, but there's a more important layer of understanding available through this divine symptom. Excess weight is a companion to industrialized nations and to third world people eating mass-produced food. It's the harbinger of a collective experiment gone wrong. It's the cure for an ignorance that would have us believe we can move as a society at a blinding pace—a speed at which it's difficult to see the results of our actions.

We create mountains of waste, produce counterfeit food, pollute our waters and atmosphere, bomb our neighbors, and behave as if the soul wounds we suffer can be dealt with by proceeding as if they don't exist. Excess weight asks us to examine how a nation of affluence can have children within its borders who starve. It begs us to look deeper at the paradox of being overfed and undernourished. It asks us to look at the hidden and heavy load that's weighing us down.

Yes, excess weight can result from eating too much and exercising too little. But these seemingly simple causes and their easy solutions are ghosts. They speak nothing as to why our behaviors are out of our control in the first place. They fail to address what ails the soul and thus prove themselves to be ineffective remedies for our deeper concerns.

Americans aren't refraining from exercise because they're lazy. Quite the contrary. We're an overworked nation. Some people don't have time to exercise; others are exhausted. Why move the body if not to celebrate it? Who really wants to exercise out of punishment and pain? Do our health clubs inspire us with their décor, their music, and their machines? Are we giving ourselves any good reasons to run and play?

Obesity and excess weight are profoundly relative. Plenty of people have what most Americans would consider too much body fat, yet those beings are happy and self-satisfied. They have a great body image, a juicy sex life, and they're healthy. There's a great debate in the research community of late that will likely continue for some time. Scientists can't decide whether or not being overweight is a disease, a symptom, a risk factor for other diseases, a nonissue that will have no ill effect on health, or perhaps even a slightly positive indicator for longevity. The answer, of course, is that carrying extra weight is all of these. The results of numerous studies continue to vary because the possibilities are truly limitless. You can be carrying around a generous amount of fat for all the right reasons, all the wrong ones, or a swirl of the two.

Depending on the study you consider, 96 to 99 percent of all people who lose weight on a weight-reducing diet gain it back within one to two years. Yet few researchers have paid attention to the small percentage who keep it off. Amazingly, what most of them have to say is that they had a significant life change—a career move, a much-needed divorce, a new love, a spiritual experience, a breakthrough sexual relationship, and so on. In other words, their stories changed, their loads were lightened, and their metabolisms transformed via the chemistry of the soul.

Sacred Nourishment

We can certainly call upon the power of the sacred in practical ways to influence the metabolism of a meal. A great place to begin is to observe how we use our spiritual power to either bless or curse.

As various authors and experts have shown us, prayer, belief, and love can cause changes locally or at a distance in people, plants, food, water, and various living organisms. We don't know exactly *how* this works but we know *that* it works. Many of us can feel when we are being "cursed" by others through judgment, slander, or gossip. We can also feel the palpable and uplifting sensations in our bodies when someone far away is cheerleading for us. These are real psychophysiological impressions that have been captured via the broadcast and reception capabilities of the heart and transduced into the chemistry of the body.

A negative self-judgment such as "I'm fat" or "I'm not beautiful" or "I am not enough as I am" is a curse. When uttered silently and continuously over time, the hex takes hold. It's a literal neurochemical instruction to the brain that is modulated by the hypothalamus, endocrine, immune, and neuropeptide networks and brought into bodily reality. It's a metabolic command sequence that can be aimed at self or other.

When we bless, we allow the Divine to pour through our heart, pumping the chemicals of affirmation and life through our vasculature. We send unseen forces into the electromagnetic field around and beyond us, and we send them nonlocally across time and space. At the very least, blessing creates a physiologic relaxation response and hence all the metabolic advantages this state offers, from increased digestive force to enhanced calorie-burning efficiency.

For these reasons, a prayer before meals makes nutritional and spiritual sense. Consider offering some special words, aloud or silent, that acknowledge the creatures and plants who offered themselves to you. Give thanks for being nourished and provided for. If making a prayer of gratitude for your food is uncomfortable for you, just add a pinch of humility. You'll find yourself more willing and considerate of Creation.

You'll experience how, by blessing your food, you're somehow blessed in return.

Yet another grounding way to embody the metabolic power of the sacred is through ritual. Most of us have daily rituals that are performed with little awareness or intention: wake up, blow nose, go to bathroom, shower, dress, drink coffee, go to work, do things. But when we invoke the Divine, the most commonplace acts are elevated. We ignite a gentle metabolic flame that burns through stagnation and circulates all manner of energy within us. Ritual, then, is the intentional calling forth of the beyond, of the unseen, the ancestors, the spirits. It confers power. It opens up a circuitry that links us with the sacred and enables the ordinary to become infused with grace.

Some of the elements that allow the power of ritual to come alive include thoughtfulness, reverence, spaciousness, openness, receptivity, gratitude, and humility. Ritual is about offering. We offer up our actions to the creative force of life. And we offer up all of who we are because, at some timeless time, all of who we are was offered to us. For many people, ritual requires a certain intellectual risk. That's because we've been taught to ignore it, to ridicule it, or we've had bad experiences with empty social and religious rituals that have left us wary of its value. But that's the past.

Perhaps the most meaningful and potent rituals are the ones we create for ourselves, in our own way and through our own intimate connection to the cosmos. What are the rituals in your life that are most meaningful? How do these rituals leave you feeling? How do they affect your body? Your energy? Your metabolism? Can you think of any activities in your life that are calling for more of your ritual attention? Consider bringing new rituals into your day if for no other reason than to experiment and notice their effects. Here are some suggestions.

Rituals of cooking: Offer gratitude as you prepare your meal. Be mindful and aware of every act—cleaning, cutting, disposing, pouring, placement. Let your reverence for food and your love of eating infuse the meal and extend to all those who dine. Slow down. Consider the beauty and timelessness of the cooking experience.

Rituals of tea or coffee: Be thoughtful, thankful, meditative, joyous—whatever qualities take you wider and deeper—as you prepare your brew. Use beautiful cups, silverware, and the like. Pause. Hold your cup with reverent intention. Infuse your drink with the Divine. Ask its special gifts to flow through your body and your day. Sip with gratitude and presence.

Rituals of offering: Upon awakening, begin your day by offering yourself to the day, to the will of the creative intelligence, to the unseen compassionate power. Offer up your body and your actions. Surrender whatever you're holding onto. Ask for a new beginning, and be willing to be that new beginning. Give yourself fully to the unknown with trust and with faith.

Rituals of medicine: Don't just swallow your vitamins, prescription pills, or painkillers—receive them. Prepare yourself to embody their gifts. Pause. Notice them. Before you ingest them, place all your pills in a small, beautiful bowl. Consciously acknowledge your reasons for taking them. Give thanks. Infuse them with the power of your belief and ask for the healing force of the unseen to operate through them purely and without harmful effects.

Rituals of beauty and hygiene: Allow for reverence, gratitude, and a sense of beauty to be present as you care for your teeth, shower or bathe, brush your hair, shave, apply makeup, polish your nails, or adorn yourself. Slow down. There's no rush. If there is, gift yourself with more time. Be aware of who you are and what you've been given. Let go of judging how the Divine Artist has crafted your form. Allow yourself to be thankful for your body and its true beauty. Let all your acts of beautifying be an offering of thanks for a gift that will someday be no more.

Sacred Foods

Have you ever had the experience of suddenly becoming attracted to a certain food or drink, consuming it often for days or weeks, and feeling convinced that despite your odd desire it was somehow a necessary medicine for you? During week 8, see whether any foods are calling to you in this way, and if they are, elevate their consumption to a sacred ritual. Acknowledge the deep wisdom of your body, trust that divine guidance can operate through your enteric nervous system, and infuse this special food with your gratitude and attention. It may be pink grapefruits that are calling you, or fresh peppermint tea, ripe blueberries, frozen corn, pickled ginger, imported chocolate, fine tequila. Whatever it is, invoke the sacred to direct you in its use and see if you can notice the subtle ways that this medicine is healing and nourishing your body.

Sacred Substances

When I was a graduate student at Sonoma State University in California, an impromptu gathering formed one evening outside a classroom building. A Native American elder was paying a visit and his friendly, open, and wise demeanor attracted a small crowd. At one point he was speaking about the sacred nature of everything in the created world. As an example he cited tobacco, which he considered to be a most sacred plant and thus one of the most powerful. At that moment a skeptical passerby happened to catch this morsel of the conversation and blurted out "I don't believe any of that 'sacred power' business about tobacco." The native elder politely turned to him with a smile and asked slowly and emphatically: "Then why do you think so many of your people are hopelessly addicted to it and destroyed by it?"

Everything has power—and that power is relative. Some businesses are more powerful than others, as are certain songs, sweeteners, computers, credit cards, laser beams, and lawn mowers. The same concept applies to food, drugs, plants, pills, or any ingestible substance. Drug companies and drug users are always searching for new and more potent substances. The same can be said for those who manufacture or consume vitamins and herbs. When we acknowledge that the power of any substance originates and issues forth from the sacred, we position ourselves to receive the greatest gifts of that substance. We are guided in its use by the hand of the unseen. We create the timeless and reverent space to let the greater intelligence speak to us. Conversely, when we fail to see the sacred here, we proceed unawares, and all manner of problems are unleashed.

Look at any challenge society is suffering around the misuse of powerful entities—drugs, alcohol, tobacco, guns—and what you're seeing is the absence of the sacred. Without the intentional invitation of the Divine into the manufacture, growing, handling, preparation, and usage of these substances, their power is transferred to the realm of the profane, which releases a poisonous chemistry and leads us down a path of destruction and despair.

Tobacco is a sacred herb to many Native people. It is used in ceremony to honor ancestors, to offer prayers sent skyward upon its smoke, and to acknowledge the interrelation between all people and all things. Every aspect of its growth, preparation, and use was made sacred and special. Tobacco addiction within Native tribes was an historically unknown concept. The white tribe took that same plant, though, engineered it to contain more addictive components, dosed it with hundreds of chemical additives, and then denied for decades its disease-forming nature, and the result is illness, addiction, and death. A sacred substance was made profane by our actions and intent.

Consider the example of sugar. If we fail to recognize its sacred nature—which, as a culture, we do—then we'll likely suffer as the dark side of its power—tooth decay, obesity, insulin resistance, diabetes, brain disease, heart disease—is exposed. Without an awareness of the sacred, we strip sugar down and produce a highly denatured version of it. We overuse it. Manufacturers pour excess amounts into their products to increase sales. Consequently, we become chemically hooked on it and blind to its effects. If you chewed on the fresh sugar cane plant every day for years, you might never see a single cavity.

Is sugar bad? Of course not. We simply need to respect it. Take a step back. Let it teach us how much is best and when enough is enough.

We've already mentioned what happens when the meat we consume is of poor quality. Truly, the ultimate factor that determines the nutritional quality of any such product is the sacred. That's because animals are sacred and the meat of animals is sacred. When we slaughter an animal, which is one of the most powerful ritual sacrifices, we are calling upon the forces of either the sacred or the profane. Without the Divine in the equation—without respect and reverence for and gratitude to the creature—we've got problems. And those kinds of problems will never be resolved with more USDA inspections. Whoever came up with the idea of "the sacred cow" knew what he or she was talking about.

What substances do you demonize? Which ones do you make sacred? Consider that every food, drug, plant, or potion is an expression of the Divine. Can you see how the sacred can offer its gifts through any substance in existence? Are you willing to see the sacred in the things you demonize? In the people you put in this category? In the qualities in yourself to which you give this charge? And can you see that all the powerful foods and drugs in our world have a simple and clear function: to serve as mirrors for us all?

Any substance can be made sacred. Even if you choose to eat something that obviously lacked a sacred connection in its growth and manufacture, we can still offer it our blessings and prayers and ask that we transmute its poisons. No thing and no one is so low that they cannot be raised up by our humanity and by the divinity that flows through us.

Of course, we'll have little interest in seeing the divine nature in food, pills, or plants if we cannot allow ourselves to see the sacred nature of our own bodies. Our science and education systems have taught us to see the body as a collection of chemicals, devoid of a Creator's hand. We think that somehow, somewhere, a long long time ago, a lifeless bunch of molecules began randomly colliding and clumping together. These meaningless collisions continued until, eons later, human beings emerged.

If you've bought into this entertaining brand of science fiction, then you likely treat your body as if it were a biological machine. You feed it, exercise it, walk it, jog it, take it for a check-up, give it a tune-up, and replace broken parts. This may work, but only to a point. Because the body is so much more than a biomechanic device, we pay the price for banishing cosmic intelligence. We find ourselves, in fact, behaving in a very unmachinelike fashion. Depression, mood swings, inner fatigue, unexplainable symptoms, and uncontrollable behavior are all signs of the soul asking to gain entrance.

So instead of searching for the next miracle diet, miracle food, or miracle supplement, consider going to the very source of the miraculous. Imagine what it would be like to see your body through the eyes of the Creator. How would a benevolent Creator look upon you? How would you look upon you if you knew your body to be a sacred vessel? How might your metabolism express itself if you held yourself in this higher light?

Week 8: Your Primary Task

This week is your opportunity to experience the metabolic power of the sacred. Your primary task is to invoke the presence of the Divine into your meals and in your relationship with your body. Commit to creating the space to allow the light of the soul to shine through during week 8 and to discovering the rich connections between your nutritional life and your spiritual world.

Exercise: The Prayer Diet

At each meal and every snack or drink you take throughout this week, without exception, offer a prayer of gratitude. No matter what the circumstance or where you are, don't miss a single serving in the prayer diet. Gently brush aside all real or imagined obstacles that would interfere with a prayerful moment. Close your eyes, release your thoughts, contact your heart, and connect to the Divine. Give thanks for the food and for anything else in your life worth being thankful for.

Invite those at the table to participate. If you eat with others who might find this uncomfortable, simply alert them that you'll be observing a moment of silence before the meal. If you have children, ask them to share aloud what they are grateful for. Notice how this changes your experience of eating and notice the effects it has on your metabolism.

Exercise: Choose Your Ritual

Refer back to the section in this chapter on sacred nourishment. Choose a ritual you'd like to focus on for the week—a ritual of cooking, tea/coffee, offering, medicine, or beauty and hygiene. Make the ritual you choose special. When enacting it, offer up your actions and thoughts to the Divine. Invoke the presence of the unseen and of the guardian beings that people your spiritual world. Allow your usual worldly approach to be elevated to a higher place. Notice what it feels like to call the energies of the sacred into your cooking, to invoke healing power into your tea, to bless your medicines and pills, or to feel the Goddess enter within as you adorn the sacred vessel you've been given. Find the quiet, gentle, magical place inside where your connection to the beyond comes alive. Notice any changes in your body, your energy level, and the quality of your vital force.

Forgiveness: The Most Potent Sacred Metabolizer

In my thirty-plus years as a nutritionist, the most powerful and life-changing strategy I've seen that liberates energy, banishes unwanted health habits, and rejuvenates the body is simply this: forgiving. I'm still amazed at how those who've had long-term eating disorders, chronic fatigue, digestive complaints, and a host of debilitating symptoms see miraculous relief when forgiving people from their past and present. If you've ever been betrayed, abused, or wounded in any way, the anger, blame, or judgment you hold is toxic. Indeed, it doesn't matter how right you are and how wrong the perpetrator is. The most poisonous chemicals on the planet are the ones we self-produce deep inside our beings. Though our poison is intended for another, it nevertheless lives within, corroding the body with acidic intent. Forgiveness heals, big time. Our most intelligent strategies in diet, exercise, medicine, and healing are ultimately ineffectual in the cloudy chemistry of the unforgiven.

Exercise: Forgiving and Healing

Take an inventory of the people in your life whom you hold responsible for some injustice. Collect on paper all the characters you still blame, still judge, and still keep hostage in your psychic prison. Be absolutely thorough in rummaging through your past and present to locate all such criminals. Include all appropriate relatives, friends, lovers, presidents, and generalized groups of people ("men," "women," "blacks," "whites," etc.). Once your list is complete, check it over to make sure it includes the three people you likely need to forgive most—your parents and yourself.

If you haven't already figured it out, your next task is to forgive everyone. This is hard work. It takes courage, and it's the most rewarding dietary strategy you could ever imagine. That's because forgiveness is a sacred metabolic act. It releases the death grip you've placed on your own cells and ignites a meta-chemistry that opens the body so that it can receive nourishment in a whole new way. Really. There's no special secret or trick to accomplishing the heroic feat of forgiveness. You just take a deep breath and do it. Dive real deep and find the soul lesson that others were helping you learn with their wounding or betraying ways. Thank them for helping you stretch to your spiritual limits and acknowledge that you are indeed a better person and have grown from their actions.

For extra credit, make a complete list of everything that remains unforgiven in you toward your parents and yourself. Note the degree of resistance you might have in doing this exercise. This is a secret indicator that the exercise is good medicine. What is it in you and in your parents that you still don't accept, that you still judge, still want to change, or still try to sweep under the rug. Once you feel complete in this inventory, compassionately love and forgive all. Acknowledge to yourself that this may be an ongoing practice, perhaps lifelong. Along the way, note the changes in your metabolism.

Exercise: Nutritional Soul Lessons

Here is your final exercise for accessing the metabolic power of the sacred. Bring your attention to any challenge with food or body that you would like to work with. This could be an illness, a symptom, a body-image concern, or a weight issue. Referring back to the section "Nutrition Lessons for the Soul," look at yourself from the perspective of the Divine and create a new and positive story as to why this issue is your "cure" rather than a "disease." How is this issue a gift from the gods? What soul lesson is it here to teach you? Expand your heart and mind as generously as possible so you can see your life from a compassionately cosmic perspective. Allow the mature wisdom of the soul to shine through so you can see yourself in a higher light. Here are some soulful thoughts on the common concerns of weight loss, depression, fatigue, and digestive health to help get you started.

Weight Loss

This is your sacred opportunity to find love for your body, to find compassion without conditions. Befriend your body. See the divinity in it. Let a higher power infuse it. Stop feeling alone in your struggle and let the grace in. Trust in your journey. Forgive yourself. See your issues with weight as a blessing, a journey you've chosen for learning some important lessons about life, lessons such as "It's not about how you look, it's about how you love." Surrender to your body as it is and love yourself exactly where you are. Perhaps you haven't lost weight because your body simply doesn't need to lose any weight and you're absolutely beautiful as you are, despite what you or anyone else has to say about it. Allow yourself to absolutely forget about losing weight, to forget about limiting yourself or punishing yourself. Take a vacation from your inner taskmaster. It's not about food or about weight. It's about you and your soul's healing. Such healing happens as we gently and sweetly inhabit our bodies in a new way. Pretend you're an angel who's just flown into your physical form to love and nurture it. Celebrate food, receive its pleasure, relax, take time for meals, and be aware of what you're doing. Begin a new and intimate relationship with food. See it as your lifeline to the pleasure and nourishment of earthly existence.

Move past vanity and tend to the soul. Slow down. Feel. Dream. Listen. Experience the darkness. Hear the voices of those who truly suffer. Speak the truth. See the hidden connections between us all. Honestly ask yourself what needs to be liberated from your being that would truly lighten you up. Would it be old anger, resentments, blame, judgments, unfinished business, unspoken words? What do you need to let go of? Who needs to be released from your life? How do you need to nourish yourself so that your body feels lovely and light rather than dense and deprived? Once you begin to *feel* lighter you train your metabolism how to *be* lighter.

Take an honest look at how long you've been at war with your body. Call for an unconditional cease-fire. Weight-loss strategies driven by fear can only fail. Even if you do lose weight through fear and self-judgment, you'll still be living in fear and self-judgment. Before you lose anything, you need to find it. It must be in your possession. If you wish to lose weight, you've got to own it. Accept it. Accept yourself. Find your center, your core, and your dignity within the whole affair. Stop being a slave to the weight-loss system. It's time to act like a queen or a king.

Create a regular eating schedule. Three meals per day is fine, five to six small meals per day is fine, two meals plus some snacks can work—it doesn't matter how you do it. Find your rhythm. Just make sure you don't starve yourself the first half of the day and then eat heavily at night. Choose a pattern and stick to it. Eat lunch. Let go of poor-quality "carbohydrate-only meals," especially at breakfast and lunch. Choose quality foods. Tune into your gut wisdom. See what you're attracted to that will grant you a healthy metabolism and a nourishing experience. Move and exercise joyously. Eliminate any aspects of working out that are cleverly disguised punishment systems. Let go of any concept of numbers, calories, points, portions, or grams. Be natural. Find your inner wisdom. Trust yourself. Be courageous in this new and uncertain journey. Have faith that you'll rebound from any challenging choices you make. Let go into the beauty of the nourishment experience. Allow your inner radiance to infuse your metabolism. Be happy now. Say good-bye to the false belief that less pounds guarantees happiness. Follow this guidance and your success is assured.

Depression

Depression is far underrated. We fail to truly honor and value it. We don't like depression, so we attempt to cast it out. But we're not meant to like depression. There's a reason for its presence that has little to do with its popularity. Depression is a visitation from the Divine. There's a message in it, perhaps many messages. Depression is a season of the soul. Is it really possible to eliminate a cold winter?

Before you medicate your depression, listen to it. If it's taken hold of you, embrace it. If you're struggling in its waters, dive in. Call upon the Divine. Pray. Rest. Feel. We have much to be depressed about. The condition of the world and the lives we lead can rightly and justly be experienced as depressing. Let's just be real about it.

It takes courage to enter into the pain of the heart. It takes a deep trust and faith to allow depression to just be. It's not an invasive demon. It's an aspect of who we are, a part of our soul life that needs a voice. It's here to rescue us. Can we listen? Can we be compassionate enough to experience all of who we are? Depression wants to help us retrieve the lost fragments of our soul. Can you enter a dark cave to find a cherished child? Can you remember your lost dreams? Can you find your innocence? Can you touch your rage? Can you rekindle your light?

The veils of depression naturally lift when we have received its gifts. If you are truly ready to let go of this visitation, oxygen is the key. Of all the research on this topic, the most consistent and successful strategy for alleviating depression is not Prozac or any medication—it's vigorous exercise. This is the time to breathe, jog, bicycle, and feel "winded." Practice breathing with meals. Nourish yourself with quality food. Rediscover the pleasure in eating. Invite the sacred into your life. Bless your depression, and bless its upliftment.

Fatigue

I've never met one person who was experiencing low energy who didn't urgently need this gift. Fatigue helps us slow down, feel, look inside, listen deeply, and make the kinds of course corrections that would otherwise go unnoticed had we not been visited by this cure. So before you look to banish your low energy, make it an honored guest. Find its message. Notice what it feels like to feel tired. Rest. Don't tell yourself you have no time to slow down and recharge. It's your life. Be honest, be brave, and make the time. No matter what the metabolic reason for your low energy, and such reasons are many, your fatigue is the soul's way to slow down your journey.

What is the real work that needs to be done? What have you been avoiding? Who are the loved ones in need of your attention? What are you giving value to that, indeed, is not so valuable after all? Where are you brilliant at fooling yourself? How do you push too hard? If you're feeling low energy, chances are you're leaking energy. Where might these leaks be? How do you disempower yourself? What places in you seem most afraid?

Issues about energy are issues about our life force and how we're using it. It's about how we're expressing or suppressing our soul's purpose. If you're doing what you want to do and what you're meant to do, you'll have plenty of energy to do it. If you're moving against the tides of the soul, against your core values, you'll secretly resist. Your body will work against itself. You'll feel tired. And you'll be attracted to eating all the wrong foods.

It's great to experiment with diet and supplements when looking to increase energy. Just know that finding your deepest inspirations will potentiate any food or substance with the force to enhance your inner fire. Living the truth of who you truly are is the key to releasing your fatigue.

Digestive Health

If you suffer from heartburn, indigestion, or fatigue after meals and if you're taking drugs to alleviate the matter, it's time to liberate yourself. This divine symptom is asking you to look closely at how you digest and assimilate life. It's alerting you that something is amiss in how you metabolize the world. Digestion is a beautiful metaphor for how we consume and process our personal affairs.

Are you moving too fast? Are you shoveling life experience into your body so quickly that there's no time to discern the proper way to break things down? Are you feeding yourself the same stale life strategies, the same patterns and habits, over and over again and confused at why you feel so ill? What beliefs do you insist on munching upon that continuously cause your gut to rebel? In what ways do you steadfastly remain unconscious, refusing to take responsibility for how your life is showing up?

Something is not working in how you live in the world, and it's not a problem with the food or your digestion. Your soul is asking you to chew on things more fully and deeply and to see how such conscious digestion of life can transform you. Be real and present with yourself. Trust that your soul can handle the things in your life that you fear are indigestible.

Approximately 80 million people in America report ongoing gastrointestinal complaints. This is neither normal nor natural. And it certainly doesn't indicate a deficiency in digestive medication.

Here's what the drug companies don't want you to know.

Most of our digestive ailments can be cured or significantly diminished by eating under the optimum state of digestion—relaxation. This secret is out in the open but few pay attention. If you've ever seen a doctor or nutritionist for digestive concerns and he or she didn't ask if you are a fast, moderate, or slow eater, didn't inquire as to the emotional-physiological state of you, the eater—whether your meals are anxious or relaxing affairs—then your practitioner has unwittingly missed the single most important determining factor of digestive well-being in all of science. Eighty million people have chronic gastrointestinal (GI) complaints because almost eighty million people are moving at high speeds. They aren't aware of what and how they eat. They've left the soul far behind in the mists.

Even if you have a bona fide digestive invader such as parasites, yeast, bacterial overgrowth, or an imbalance in stomach acidity, you'll still never achieve full relief and digestive healing, no matter what pills or medications you're prescribed, until you round out your metabolic picture by creating a healing digestive milieu. That means creating parasympathetic dominance through relaxed eating. It means listening to the soul lessons that your digestion is teaching you—practicing the principles of breathing, relaxation, awareness, and pleasure. Slow down, even within your hectic schedule, and land in your body. Nourish yourself.

Many people with ongoing GI complaints have locked their systems into chronic sympathetic activation. It may take only several days to undo this; then again, it may take several months of focused practice to release the grip of this metabolic vice. Even if you forever have a sensitive digestive system, consider this to be your friend, a faithful barometer that always lets you know when you're too far ahead of yourself or not listening to your inner wisdom.

Pay special attention to attuning to your ENS intelligence, your gut wisdom, seeking its advice on food choices. Oftentimes, gastrointestinal complaints directly result from combinations of food that are incompatible with our physiology. Access this information by slowing down, tuning in, and asking the question "What would nourish me?" Then act upon the answer. Thank your gut for being a wonderfully alert system that sounds the alarm when your style of eating and living is out of sync with the rhythms of heart and soul.

Key Lessons

- Our connection to the sacred can access little understood yet potent metabolic changes.

- Love, truth, courage, commitment, compassion, forgiveness, faith, surrender, and other sacred qualities are potent metabolic enhancers.

- When life is calling these qualities from us, they act as healing catalysts in the body.

- We have the power to "bless" or "curse," thus affecting energetically and nonlocally our food, our selves, and our fellow humans.

- Ritual accesses the meta-chemistry of the sacred.

- When we treat a food, drug, or the body as "profane," the chemistry of pain and confusion is released. Treating these as sacred reveals a healing and transformational chemistry.

- The cure for our metabolic ills are often found within the heart of those very challenges. Indeed, the illness is the cure.

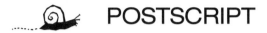 POSTSCRIPT

Your Metabolic Journey

Metabolism isn't something we fix. You can measure certain aspects of it, yet metabolism itself is measureless. You can tweak certain parts of it, yet it remains always whole. You can command it to do your bidding, yet it will always answer to a higher source.

Metabolism is not a thing. It's a journey.

It is an ever-moving, ever-changing ocean of chemistry whose depths are unfathomable and whose ways are predictably unpredictable. Metabolism ebbs and flows with the rhythms of the world and moves to the music of the spheres. It is an epic poem and an infinite symphony. It is at once a current and a currency. It is the downstream waters of the Divine. Metabolism can cause events to happen, but it is itself an effect. It is the effect of your life, your existence, your soul. It is a mirror image of your sacred form, the material portal for cosmic forces, a momentary abode for your eternal spirit.

The way we navigate through our metabolic journey is the way we navigate through our life journey. In other words, how you treat your body—how you nourish it, feed it, exalt it, or dethrone it—is the way you treat yourself. If your body is seen as special, then you'll see your life as special. If your metabolism is seen as a chaotic, frightening void, then life will feel the same way too. If you invite toxicity into the body then you are asking it into your personal world. If you choose to not see how your style of living creates your health, then you are choosing to not see how your choices create your reality. If you invite the sacred into your personal world, you will find it inhabiting your metabolic world.

This is all good news. That's because you can change how you do life at any moment in time and in doing so you can transform your biology. As with all journeys that have been described by the great poets, playwrights, and storytellers throughout the ages, your metabolic journey takes you through magical lands, strange terrains, dangerous places, dark forests, sacred mountaintops, markets, carnivals, circus tents, the healer's sanctuary, the garden of delights, the abyss. You'll find charlatans dressed in expert's clothes, experts costumed like clowns, shamans in business suits, buddhas in bikinis, and allies giggling at you in the most unsuspecting guises, hiding everywhere.

Begin your metabolic journey now.

Allow your body and your outlook to be new again. Let the journey be what it is, because that's what it will be anyway. When uncertainty reigns, let it be your guide. When your inner knowing issues forth, follow it with trust and self-respect. When your metabolism is wounded, let it cry. Before you test the chemistry of your body, taste your tears. Before you take a drug, meditate, reflect, and pray. Before you limit yourself with a diet, expand yourself with love. Before you lose a pound, gain an insight. Before you exercise, be still. Before you attempt to cast out a bad habit, thank it for its teachings. Before you harm yourself in thought, word, or deed, pause. Before you allow someone dominion over your body, awaken. Before you seek advice, remember your wisdom. Before you speak, make sure it's an improvement on silence. Before you're intimate with another, touch the sacred. Before you fall ill, catch yourself. Before you lapse into fear, choose light. Before you believe in a world absent of a Creator, give birth. Before you remember your divine purpose, celebrate its imminent arrival. Before you eat, give gratitude. Before you sit for long hours, dance. Before you arise, bless everything. Before you sleep, do the same. Before you live another day, agree to be here in your fullness. And before you breathe another breath, choose eternity, choose love, choose now.

The Institute for the Psychology of Eating

Marc David founded The Institute for the Psychology of Eating, an educational organization unlike any other. The Institute is on a mission to forever change the way the world understands food, body, and health. They offer trainings for professionals, programs for the public, online events, live workshops and conferences as well as plenty of free online content and inspiration. Their premier professional offering, the eating psychology coach certification training, teaches students to work with the most common and compelling eating challenges of our times— weight, body image, overeating, binge eating, emotional eating, endless dieting, and nutrition-related health challenges that have an emotional component such as digestion, fatigue, mood, immunity, and others. The Institute is the worlds first and only teaching organization dedicated to a forward thinking, positive, holistic approach to eating psychology. Their students, friends, and tribe come from all walks of life and many different countries with this one common goal—to learn a better way to heal our relationship with food, body, planet, and soul. It's time for a fresh, new approach. It's time to find real and lasting relief from our eating challenges, and to finally discover a relationship with food and body that's truly nourishing and empowering. Please join the Institute in a new movement that's making a real difference in the world.

Learn more at psychologyofeating.com

Notes

Week 1: *The Metabolic Power of Relaxation*

1. My sources for this chart on the effects of the stress response are as follows:

A. Hanck, "Stress and Vitamin Deficiency," *International Journal for Vitamin and Nutrition Research* 26 (1984).

S. Porta, "Interactions Between Magnesium and Stress Hormones in Stress," *Mengen und Spurenelemente* (December 1991).

R. A. Anderson, "Stress Effects on Chromium Nutrition," Proceedings of Alltech's Tenth Annual Symposium (Nottingham University Press, 1994).

A. Singh, "Biochemical Indices of Selected Trace Minerals: Effect of Stress," *American Journal of Clinical Nutrition* 67, no. 1 (1991). This study documents decreased levels of zinc, iron, and selenium in men under stress.

N. Mei, "Role of the Autonomic Nervous System in the Regulation of Transit, Absorption and Storage of Nutrients," *Reproduction, Nutrition, Development* 26, no. 5B (1986) (France).

G. A. Bray, "The Nutrient Balance Hypothesis: Peptides, Sympathetic Activity, and Food Intake," *Annals of The New York Academy of Sciences* 676 (March 15, 1993).

W. J. Kort, "The Effect of Chronic Stress on the Immune Response," *Advances in Neuroimmunology* 4, no. 1 (1994).

J. D. Soderholm, "Stress and the Gastrointestinal Tract," *American Journal of Physiology* 280, no. 1 (January 2001).

G. Aguilera, "The Renin Angiotensin System and the Stress Response," *Annals of The New York Academy of Sciences* 771 (December 29, 1995).

D. Pignatelli, "Direct Effect of Stress on Adrenocortical Function," *Hormone Metabolism Research* 30, no. 6/7 (June/July 1998).

J. L. Cuevas, "Spontaneous Swallowing Rate and Emotional State," *Digestive Diseases and Sciences* 40, no. 2 (February 1995).

J. E. Dimsdale, "Variability of Plasma Lipids in Response to Emotional Arousal," *Psychosomatic Medicine* 44, no. 5 (1982).

S. Kaplan, "Effects of Cortisol on Amino Acid in Skeletal Muscle and Plasma," *Endocrinology* 72 (February 1963).

P. Havel, "The Contribution of the Autonomic Nervous System to Changes of Glucagons and Insulin Secretion During Hypoglycemic Stress," *Endocrine Reviews* 10, no. 3 (August 1989).

Hans Selye, *The Stress of Life* (New York: Van Nostrand, 1984). This is the classic work on the physiology of the stress response.

2. P. Bjorntorp, "Psychosocial Factors and Fat Distribution," *Obesity in Europe '91* (Proceedings of the 3rd European Congress on Obesity, 1992). This is an excellent research paper on obesity and stress.

E. T. Poehlman, "Sympathetic Nervous System Activity, Body Fatness, and Body Fat Distribution in Younger and Older Males," *Journal of Applied Physiology* 78, no. 3 (March 1995).

S. Knox, "Biobehavioral Mechanisms in Lipid Metabolism and Atherosclerosis: An Overview," *Metabolism: Clinical and Experimental* 42, no. 9 (suppl. 1) (September 1993).

B. G. Lipinski, "Life Change Events as Correlates of Weight Gain," *Recent Advances in Obesity Research* (Proceedings of the First International Congress on Obesity, London, 1975).

J. Istvan, "Body Weight and Psychological Distress in NHANES I," *International Journal of Obesity* 21, no. 5 (October 1992).

3. T. E. Burkovskaya, "Kinetics of Elemental Content Changes of Bone Tissue of Mice During Evolution of Hypokinetic Stress," *Biological Trace Element Research* 43–45, (Fall 1994) (Moscow).

4. D. Michelson, "Bone Mineral Density in Women with Depression," *The New England Journal of Medicine* 335, no. 16, (October 17, 1996).

5. Melvyn Werbach, *Nutritional Influences on Illness* (Tarzana, Calif.: Third Line Press, 1993). For a good list of resources on this topic, see the section on osteoporosis.

Other resources for this chapter include:

R. Forster and R. Estabrook, "Is Oxygen an Essential Nutrient?" *Annual Review of Nutrition* 13 (1993).

C. R. Honig, "Oxygen Transport and Its Interaction with Metabolism: A Systems View of Aerobic Capacity" *Medical Science and Sports Exercise* 24, no. 1 (January 1992).

D. L. Gilbert, *Oxygen and Living Processes: An Interdisciplinary Approach* (New York: Springer-Verlag, 1981).

H. Weiner, *Perturbing the Organism: The Biology of Stressful Experience* (University of Chicago Press, 1992).

Robert Sapolsky, *Why Zebras Don't Get Ulcers* (New York: W. H. Freeman, 1994).

Week 2: The Metabolic Power of Quality

1. Weston A. Price, *Nutrition and Physical Degeneration* (New Canaan, Conn.: Keats Publishing, 2003). This is the classic work on the dramatic differences in health between those on traditional diets versus commercial/industrial diets.

2. For convincing evidence of the health harms of high protein from meat, refer to *The Food Revolution* by John Robbins (Boston: Conari Press, 2000). For convincing evidence on the other side, see H. Spencer, *American Journal of Clinical Nutrition* 37, no. 6 (June 1983), June 1983 and S. Fallon, *Price-Pottenger Nutrition Foundation Health Journal,* 1996.

3. A. Lopez, "Some Interesting Relationships between Dietary Carbohydrates and Serum Cholesterol," *American Journal of Clinical Nutrition* 18, no. 2 (February 1966).

Other resources for this chapter include:

A. K. Kant, "Consumption of Energy-Dense, Nutrient-Poor Foods by the U.S. Population: Effect on Nutrient Profiles," *Journal of the American College of Nutrition* 72, no. 4 (October 2000).

E. Gunderson, "FDA Total Diet Study, July 1986–April 1991: Dietary Intake of Pesticides, Selected Elements, and Other Chemicals," *Journal of AOAL International* 78, no. 6 (November–December 1995).

"Food Safety and Quality as Affected by Organic Farming," in *UN Food and Agriculture Report,* July 2000.

"Organic Foods vs. Supermarket Foods: Elemental Levels," in *Journal of Applied Nutrition* 45 (1993).

"Exposure to Pesticides Lowered When Young Children Go Organic, Researchers Determine," *New York Times,* March 25, 2003.

Paula Baillie-Hamilton, *The Body Restoration Plan: Eliminate Chemical Calories and Repair Your Body's Natural Slimming System* (New York: Avery Publishing, 2003).

M. Alice Ottoboni, *The Dose Makes the Poison* (New York: Van Nostrand, 1991).

Russell Blaylock, *Excitotoxins: The Taste that Kills* (New Mexico: Health Press, 1996).

Sandra Steingraber, *Living Downstream* (New York: Vintage Books, 1998).

Richard Gerber, *Vibrational Medicine,* (Rochester, Vt.: Bear & Company, 1988).

Week 3: The Metabolic Power of Awareness

1. S. A. Giduck, "Cephalic Reflexes: Their Role in Digestion and Possible Roles in Absorption and Metabolism," *Journal of Nutrition* 117, no. 7 (July 1987).

2. G. R. Barclay, "Effect of Psychosocial Stress on Salt and Water Transport in

the Human Jejunum," *Gastroenterology* 93, no. 1 (July 1987).

3. B. Baldaro, "Effects of an Emotional Negative Stimulus on Cardiac, Electro-gastrographic, and Respiratory Responses," *Perceptual and Motor Skills* 71, no. 2 (October 1990).

4. T. L. Powley, "Diet and Cephalic Phase Insulin Responses," *American Journal of Clinical Nutrition* 14, no. 4 (September 1985).

5. J. Furness and J. Bornstein, "The Enteric Nervous System and Its Extrinsic Connections," in *Textbook of Gastroenterology* (Philadelphia: Lippincott, 1995).

6. Michael Gershon, *The Second Brain* (New York: Perennial, 1999).

7. T. E. Adrian and S. R. Bloom, "The Effect of Food on Gut Hormones," *Advances in Food and Nutrition Research* 37 (1993*).

8. Sandra Blakeslee, "Complex and Hidden Brain in the Gut Makes Cramps, Butterflies, and Valium," *New York Times,* January 23, 1996.

Other resources for this chapter include:

S. McCrae, "Changes in pattern of fasting jejunal motor activity during mental stress," *Journal of Physiology* 308 (1980).

M. Costa, "The Enteric Nervous System," *The American Journal of Gastroenterology* 89, no. 8 (1994).

S. Wolf, "The Stomach's Link to the Brain," *Federation Proceedings* 44, no. 14 (1985).

R. K. Goyal, "The Enteric Nervous System," *The New England Journal of Medicine* 334, no. 17 (April 25, 1996).

L. Johnson, *Gastrointestinal Physiology* (Philadelphia: Mosby, 1991).

Raphael Kellman, *Gut Reactions* (New York: Broadway Books, 2002).

Week 4: The Metabolic Power of Rhythm

1. C. A. Czeisler, "Stability, Precision, and Near-24-Hour Period of the Human Pacemaker," *Science* 284 (June 25, 1999).

2. David Lloyd, *Ultradian Rhythms in Life Processes* (New York: Springer-Verlag, 1992).
   Providers Manual—Clinical Training in Mind/Body Medicine, Harvard Mind/Body Medical Institute 1995.

3. T. W. Uhde, "Caffeine: Relationship to Human Anxiety, Plasma MHPG, and Cortisol," *Psychopharmacology Bulletin* 20, no. 3 (1984).

4. T. S. Wiley, *Lights Out* (New York: Pocket Books, 2000).

Other resources for this chapter include:

E. M. Berry, "Foods and Their Effects on Sleep Patterns," *International Clinical Nutrition Review* 7, no. 2 (1987).

A. Concu, "Indirect Evidence in Humans of Nervous Parasympathetic Predominance in Integrated Responses to a Balanced Meal," *Medical Science Research* 20, no. 19 (1992) (Italy).

E. L. Gibson, "Increased Salivary Cortisol Reliably Induced by a Protein-Rich Midday Meal," *Psychosomatic Medicine* 61, no. 2 (1999).

F. Brouns, "Is the Gut an Athletic Organ? Digestion, Absorption and Exercise" *Sports Medicine* 15, no. 4 (1993).

H. M. Lloyd, "Mood and Cognitive Performance Effect of Isocaloric Lunches Differing in Fat and Carbohydrate Content," *Physiology and Behavior* 56, no. 1 (July 1994).

B. C. Johnson, "Nutrient Intake as a Time Signal for Circadian Rhythm," *American Institute of Nutrition* 122, no. 9 (April 28, 1992).

P. J. Rogers, "Nutrition and Mental Performance," *Proceedings of the Nutrition Society* 53, no. 2 (1994).

Kenneth Rose, *The Body in Time* (New York: Wiley and Sons, 1988).

A. Reinberg *Introduction to Chronobiology* (New York: Springer-Verlag, 1983).

A. T. Winfree, *The Timing of Biological Clocks* (New York: Scientific American Books, 1987).

LifeWaves International: www.lifewaves.com. This website features the unique work of Dr. Irv Dardik.

Week 5: The Metabolic Power of Pleasure

1. This report was delivered by Margo Denke of the Center for Human Nutrition, University of Texas Health Science Center, at the annual meeting of the American Heart Association, 1987.
2. "Food that Tastes Good Is More Nutritious," reported in *Tufts University Health and Nutrition Letter,* October 2000.
3. Guy Murchie, *The Seven Mysteries of Life* (Boston: Houghton Mifflin, 1978).
4. T. D. Geracioti, "Meal-Related Cholecystokinin Secretion in Eating and Affective Disorders," *Pharmacology Bulletin* 25, no. 3 (1989) and J. Hirsch, "A Clinical Perspective on Peptides and Food Intake," *American Journal of Clinical Nutrition* 55, no. 1 (1992).
5. M. M. Hetherton, "Pleasure and Excess: Liking For and Over-consumption of Chocolate," *Physiology and Behavior* 57, no. 1 (1995).

Other resources for this chapter include

A. Levine, "Opioids—Are They Regulators of Feeding?" *Annals of the New York Academy of Sciences* 575 (1989).

J. C. Melchior, "Palatability of a Meal Influences Release of Beta-Endorphin and of Potential Regulators of Food Intake in Healthy Human Subjects," *Appetite* 22, no. 3 (June 1994).

G. A. Bray, "Peptides Affect the Intake of Specific Nutrients and the Sympathetic Nervous System," *American Journal of Clinical Nutrition* 55, no. 1 (January 1992).

J. E. Blundell, "Regulation of Nutrient Supply: the Brain and Appetite Control," *Proceedings of the Nutrition Society* 53, no. 2 (July 1994).

J. E. Blundell, "Serotonin and the Biology of Feeding," *American Journal of Clinical Nutrition* 55, no. 1 (January 1992).

G. P. Smith, "The Satiety Effect of Cholecystokinin: Recent Program and Current Problems," *Annals of the New York Academy of Sciences* 448 (1985).

"Discovering Something New in Food: Pleasure," *New York Times,* December 30, 1992.

G. J. Dockray, *Gut Peptides: Biochemistry and Physiology* (Edinburgh: Churchill Livingstone, 1994).

R. Ornstein and D. Sobel, *Healthy Pleasures* (New York: Da Capo Press/Perseus Publishing, 1990).

Week 6: The Metabolic Power of Thought

1. Ernest Rossi, *The Psychobiology of Mind-Body Healing* (New York: Norton, 1986). This book offers some excellent science, insights, and diagrams regarding the mind-body connection.
2. J. W. Fielding, "Adjunct Chemotherapy in Operable Gastric Cancer," *World Journal of Surgery* 7, no. 3 (1983).
3. "Placebo—The Hidden Asset in Healing" in *Investigations,* Institute of Noetic Sciences Research Bulletin 2, no. 14 (1985).
4. D. S. Moore, *Statistics: Concepts and Controversies* (New York: Freeman, 1995).
5. S. B. Penick, "The effect of expectation on response to phenmetrazine," *Psychosomatic Medicine* 26, no. 4 (1964).
6. Kenneth Cooper, *The Antioxidant Revolution* (Nashville: Thomas Nelson, 1994).

Other resources for this chapter include:

R. L. Shames, "Nutritional Management of Stress-Induced Dysfunction," *Applied Nutritional Science Reports 2002,* Advanced Nutrition Publications Inc., available through the Institute for Functional Medicine.

R. Ornstein and D. Sobel, *The Healing Brain* (New York: Simon and Schuster, 1988).

Norman Cousins, *The Healing Heart* (New York: Norton, 1983).

Henry Dreher, *The Immune Power Personality* (New York: Penguin, 1996).

Howard Brody, *The Placebo Response* (New York: Harper Collins, 2000).

Larry Dossey, *Recovering the Soul* (New York: Bantam, 1989).

Blair Justice, *Who Gets Sick* (Los Angeles: Tarcher, 1987).

Week 7: The Metabolic Power of Story

1. "Multiple Personality—Mirrors of a New Model of Mind?" *Investigations,* Institute of Noetic Sciences Research Bulletin 1, no 3/4.
2. B. G. Braun, "Psychophysiologic Phenomena in Multiple Personality," *American Journal of Clinical Hypnosis* 26, no. 2 (1983). This report also lists other examples of multiple personality disorder patients expressing allergies in specific personalities.

Other resources for this chapter include:

Brendan O'Regan and Rick Carlson, "Defining Health: The State of the Art," *Holistic Health Review* 3, no. 2 (1979).

A. Ziegler, *Archetypal Medicine* (New York: Continuum International Publishing, 2000).

James Hillman, *Healing Fiction* (Barrytown, N. Y.: Station Hill Press, 1983).

Larry Dossey, *Meaning and Medicine* (New York: Bantam, 1991).

Lynn Payer, *Medicine and Culture* (New York: Henry Holt, 1988).

Week 8: The Metabolic Power of the Sacred
Resources for this chapter include:

"Asking if Obesity Is a Disease or Just a Symptom," *New York Times,* April 16, 2002.

"God and the Brain: How We're Wired for Spirituality," *Newsweek,* May 7, 2001.

Joseph Chilton Pearce, *The Biology of Transcendence* (Rochester, Vt.: Park Street Press, 2002).

Michael Murphy, *The Future of the Body* (Los Angeles: Tarcher, 1992).

Larry Dossey, *Healing Beyond the Body* (Boston: Shambhala, 2001).

Larry Dossey, *Healing Words* (New York: HarperCollins, 1993).

Dean Ornish, *Love and Survival* (New York: Harper Collins, 1997).

Sandra Ingerman, *Medicine for the Earth* (New York: Three Rivers Press, 2000).

Eugene d'Aquili, *The Mystical Mind: Probing the Biology of Religious Experience* (Minneapolis: Fortress Press, 1999).

Robin Robertson, *The Sacred Kitchen* (Novato, Calif.: New World Library, 1999).

James Hillman, *The Soul's Code* (New York: Random House, 1996.

Bibliography

Barks, Coleman. *The Illuminated Rumi*. New York: Broadway Books, 1997.

Buck, William. *Mahabharata*. Berkeley: University of California Press, 1973.

Brody, Howard. *The Placebo Response*. New York: HarperCollins, 2000.

Calasso, Roberto. *Ka: Stories of the Mind and Gods of India*. New York: Vintage 1998.

Dossey, Larry. *Healing Beyond the Body*. Boston: Shambhala Publications, 2001.

———. *Meaning and Medicine*. New York: Bantam Books, 1991.

———. *Recovering the Soul*. New York: Bantam Books, 1989.

———. *Reinventing Medicine*. San Francisco: HarperCollins, 1999.

Fallon, Sally. *Nourishing Traditions*. Washington, D.C.: New Trends Publishing, 1999.

Hillman, James. *Healing Fiction*. Barrytown, N.Y.: Station Hill Press, 1983.

———. *Re-Visioning Psychology*. New York: Harper & Row, 1975.

———. *The Soul's Code*. New York: Random House, 1996.

Holmes, Ernest. *The Science of Mind*. New York: Tarcher, 1998.

Hyman, Mark, and Liponis, Mark. *Ultra-Prevention*. New York: Scribner, 2003.

Lao Tzu. *Tao Te Ching*. New York: Concord Grove Press, 1983.

Levine, Peter. *Waking the Tiger*. Berkeley, Calif.: North Atlantic Books, 1997.

Murchie, Guy. *The Seven Mysteries of Life*. Boston: Houghton Mifflin, 1978.

Murphy, Michael. *The Future of the Body*. Los Angeles: Tarcher, 1992.

Ottoboni, Alice. *The Dose Makes the Poison*. New York: Van Nostrand Reinhold, 1991.

Payer, Lynn. *Medicine and Culture*. New York: Henry Holt, 1988.

Pearsall, Paul. *The Heart's Code*. New York: Broadway Books, 1998.

Pearce, Joseph Chilton. *The Biology of Transcendence*. Rochester, Vt.: Park Street Press, 2002.

Pollan, Michael. *The Botany of Desire*. New York: Random House, 2001.

Ravnskov, Uffe. *The Cholesterol Myths*. Washington, D.C.: New Trends Publishing, 2000.

Robbins, John. *The Food Revolution*. Boston: Conari Press, 2001.

Rosenthal, Joshua. *The Energy Balance Diet*. Indianapolis: Alpha Books, 2003.

Rossi, Ernest. *The Psychobiology of Mind-Body Healing*. New York: Norton, 1986.

Sapolsky, Robert. *Why Zebras Don't Get Ulcers*. New York: W. H. Freeman, 1994.

Tolle, Eckhart. *The Power of Now*. Novato, Calif.: New World Library, 1999.

Schmidt, Gerhard. *The Dynamics of Nutrition*. Rhode Island: Bio-Dynamic Literature, 1987.

———. *The Essentials of Nutrition*. Rhode Island: Bio-Dynamic Literature, 1987.

Shealy, Norman, and Myss, Caroline. *The Creation of Health*. Walpole, N.H.: Stillpoint Publications, 1993.

Werbach, Melvyn. *Nutritional Influences on Illness*. Tarzana, Calif.: Third Line Press, 1993.

Wiley, T. S. *Lights Out*. New York: Pocket Books, 2000.